LONE STAR LEGACY

The Birth of Group Hospitalization
and The Story of Blue Cross and
Blue Shield of Texas

Samuel Schaal

P.O. Box 655730

Dallas, Texas 75265

ISBN: 1-884363-17-2

Library of Congress Cataloging-in-Publication Data

Schaal, Samuel, 1952-
    Lone Star legacy : the birth of group hospitalization and the story of Blue Cross and Blue Shield of Texas / by Samuel Schaal.
      p. cm.
    ISBN 1-884363-17-2
    1. Blue Cross and Blue Shield of Texas. 2. Insurance, Health—Texas. 3. Insurance, Hospitalization—Texas. I. Title.

HG9398.B58 S33 1999
368.38'2'0065764—dc21
                                      99-052361

Manufactured in the United States using acid-free paper
Published by Odenwald Press
Printed by Taylor Publishing, Dallas, Texas
Cover design by Al Carnley
Page design by Wright Type Company, Dallas, Texas

"WHAT WE DO FOR OURSELVES
DIES WITH US —
WHAT WE DO FOR OTHERS
REMAINS AND IS IMMORTAL"

Table of Contents

Foreword

Rogers K. Coleman, M.D.
Chairman of the Board
Health Care Service Corporation
Texas Division President

The legacy of an organization is a story about its people. The people who have been Blue Cross and Blue Shield of Texas throughout this distinguished legacy have been, for the most part, unusually dedicated individuals who joined the company because it was more than a "job." They had a sense of mission, a passion for doing good things for others. That passion contained a customer focus and empathy, best exemplified by a motivating sign around the company in recent years with the caption "Picture yourself as the customer."

This was likely inherited from the old Baylor Plan in Dallas, which was the founding of the Blue Cross idea in this nation. This focus on the customer and our special relationship with health care professionals has been part of our legacy. It has carried forward to this day. The people of Blue Cross and Blue Shield of Texas know that there is no quality in health benefits unless there is a special relationship with those who deliver the care to the sick and injured and who seek to help in preventing illness and injury among those who have our coverage. Such is the nature of this legacy.

It has been our privilege to have served all segments of the market in Texas. We have concentrated on serving businesses, large and small. We have had unusually large involvement in covering the employees of schools, municipalities and other governmental entities. We were the original contractors for the Medicaid program in Texas and for the Medicare program, expanding eventually to serve Medicare beneficiaries in multiple areas throughout the United States. We have served the Federal Employee Program since its inception, and we have served the State of Texas employees most of the time since their Uniform Group Insurance Program was initiated. We have had unusual concern for those who have no health benefit coverage, and we have supported legislation to help solve the problem of the uninsured. We have supported with our work and our money the Caring For Children Foundation of Texas, Inc., providing benefits for children who otherwise would have no coverage. "We" have been and are the people of Blue Cross and Blue Shield of Texas. Such is the nature of this legacy.

There are two things to keep in mind about the story you are about to read. First, history is the ultimate judge of success or failure. I speak for thousands of present and past associates at the company when I express pride in being among those who served throughout this legacy. Whatever history's ultimate judgment, we have known good and passionate people who have worked to serve those who had a relationship with our organization. And we are grateful for the opportunity.

Second, there are always leaders who are best remembered, and they are worthy of all the honor bestowed upon them. Yet those remembered leaders could not have accomplished all that has been done by themselves. No one person, nor even a few persons, can rightfully accept credit for great accomplishments. Leaders establish direction, and they are able to give authority for actions. Accomplishments occur when thousands of associates catch a vision and a mission and invest their time and talents to bring about amazing results that make leaders look like, perhaps, geniuses and heroes. To the extent we have been successful, and only history can judge that, it is largely due to the good work of many individuals. Depicting all of the diversity present in Texas, those individuals have each brought strength and unique advantages to the workforce, and these have contributed to whatever success we have accomplished in this legacy.

There have been times in this story when we have failed. These have been failures in judgment, often arising from zeal to do things too quickly. Hopefully, dispassionate history will show that we learned from those failures, and those lessons have made us better able to do that which has been our passion—to serve our customers better every day. Such is the nature of this legacy.

On December 31, 1998, after more than three years of discussions and a prolonged legal encounter, Blue Cross and Blue Shield of Texas merged with Health Care Service Corporation (HCSC), a Mutual Legal Reserve Company in Illinois. HCSC is the Blue Cross and Blue Shield

Plan in Illinois. At this writing it is apparent that the good reasons for the merger are being accomplished:

- The Texas Plan needed a new information technology platform. The Blue Chip system has met or exceeded our expectations.

- To compete in a consolidating industry, the Texas Plan needed additional financial strength. The merger brings that added financial strength.

- The Texas Plan needed additional expertise in its HMO business. HCSC has that expertise.

- The Illinois Plan needed geographic diversity and additional market potential. The merger brings those features.

- Both Plans were looking for a merger partner with similar culture, mission and aspirations for the future. Both Plans found those characteristics.

The merger and the integration of the two Plans into one company have gone very well. Our board of directors, our senior management, our staff officers, directors, managers and almost ten thousand associates are well along in arriving at the goal of one company serving almost six million members, balancing additional growth with financial strength.

We have begun a new era in our legacy.

Acknowledgments

The third time, they say, is the charm. This story of Blue Cross and Blue Shield of Texas is the third such attempt but the first to be actually published.

In 1964 a public relations firm was hired to write the company history and the result was a short, breezy and perhaps overly heroic recitation of company events. The resulting work was not published. In late 1975 Tom Beauchamp, then president of the company, asked Harley West, the retired vice president of marketing, if he would write a history of the company. West considered himself more of an archivist than a writer, and he produced a draft impressive in its detail, compiled chiefly from board minutes and personal memories. He took the history of the company up through 1960. It was prepared primarily for the archives as a record rather than a popular history to be actually read.

In 1994 I resigned as director of public information to pursue graduate studies in theology and continued part-time employment with the company. Carolyn Colley said that the board had long wanted her to have a history of the company written. We began charting plans for organizing the company archives, interviewing some retired and active employees, and writing the book. I began actual writing in early 1998. My goal was to produce a history that was readable and reflective of the human stories that have been a part of this company.

That the story of the company has finally seen print after several efforts is due in part to the merger with Blue Cross and Blue Shield of Illinois. The merger presented a good occasion for publication since it tells the story of the Texas Plan as an autonomous entity, up to the merger on December 31, 1998.

That even the best individual effort is in reality an effort of many is exemplified by the book you hold in your hands. I am indebted to many people for this work:

For generous assistance in hours of interviews, my special thanks to the people who related stories not otherwise captured in the company archives, giving this story its color and character: Gene Aune, Jack Buzbee, Rogers Coleman, M.D., Annie Laurie Drews, Elaine Gwaltney, Walt Hachmeister, E.W. Hahn, Barbara Harvey, Judy Johnson, John Justin, Vernon Walker, George Walters and Lelia Wright.

For assistance in general research: Marilyn Mathis, Barbara Raley and Kirk Freeman. For answering many "do you remember when...." questions at the spur of the moment: Greg Moore.

For administrative assistance: Marilyn "Mimi" Speckmann, Pat Johnson, Pat Hefko, Sherry Mealy, Vicki Hawkins, Lonnie Tutson and Darlene Kie.

For creative assistance: Mary Jo Beebe, who served as my editor, and Al Carnley, who designed the cover art.

For help in reviewing portions of the manuscript: Marilyn Mathis, Carolyn Colley, Gary Fritzsche and Rogers Coleman, M.D. Especially I want to thank Jean Perkins, whose careful eye caught many errors. She also tended the list of board members in the appendix.

For valuable aid in proofing, Cray Pixley, Janice Mauren and Jean Perkins.

For helping me to manage the project successfully: Carolyn Colley (now retired) and Teresa Sheffield.

For all these people I am grateful, but I remain responsible for the content of this book and any errors it may contain.

I dedicate this work to the pioneering spirit of Blue Cross and Blue Shield of Texas and the ongoing success of Health Care Service Corporation, being the merged company of the Texas and Illinois Plans. HCSC now holds the "Lone Star Legacy" in its history and it is my prayer that this book contributes to our present understanding of ourselves (and the possibilities of our future) by first understanding our heritage.

Samuel Schaal
Richardson, Texas
July 1999

Part One

The Birth of Group Hospitalization

1 | 1929: The Man and the Formula

"I have been studying your actuarial data and our hospital records for many weeks and submit this plan to the teachers of Dallas, confident that to none will the plan prove a burden, but on the other hand a blessing to many in the hour of pain and stress."
Justin Ford Kimball

He agreed to the task when he was approaching his fifty-seventh year—an age when most people contemplated retirement and a gentle easing out of active life. His professional career had been filled with remarkable accomplishments, and he was well known in the flourishing city of Dallas, rubbing elbows with the elite citizens of that community. It was perhaps his local reputation as a no-nonsense man of innovative accomplishments that drew the interest toward hiring him for the challenge.

The man was Justin Ford Kimball, and the task was restoring Baylor University Hospital in Dallas to financial health. The year was 1929, but the stock market had not yet crashed, and the rest of the nation was still riding high on expectations of an ever-expanding economy. Though Baylor Hospital's fiscal troubles were not caused by the Great Depression, that cataclysmic event would intensify concern about the hospital's finances.

Kimball agreed to the task reluctantly, for he insisted that he was more of a "school man" than a "hospital man." It is fortunate that he agreed because what he did was much more than stabilize the finances of one hospital. His simple idea began a movement first known as "group hospitalization" and later as the national System of Blue Cross and Blue Shield Plans. Also, his idea would help create the marketplace demand for health insurance to which the commercial insurance companies would finally respond after long denying the actuarial possibility of such a product.

What we know today as the sprawling health care industry, with hospitals and physicians and many forms of high-technology medical miracles, was just beginning to take form in the 1920s. How to finance this growing system was a burning topic of the day. No one had yet arrived at a practical answer.

The man

Justin Ford Kimball was born on Sunday, August 25, 1872. He was the only child of Justin A. Kimball, a Baptist minister and college professor and Elizabeth Ford Kimball, who died when he was only about a year old. His father later remarried and in that union had another son and a daughter.

Young Justin was raised in the East Texas town of Mineola. His life as a scholar started almost as soon as he could walk. He says his father taught him Latin "when I was not much out of my infancy" and Greek and Hebrew a little later. In his senior years, Kimball quipped that his father wanted to teach him such difficult subjects because he wanted his son to learn to keep his mouth shut in five different languages.

When it was time for Justin to attend college, his father took a position as professor of Greek and theology at Mount Lebanon College in Louisiana, enrolled his son at the college and taught him Greek in the classroom along with other students. Even before Justin achieved his bachelor's degree at Mount Lebanon, he was pressed into service as a teacher in the surrounding Louisiana countryside. He graduated from Mount Lebanon in 1890 and for two years continued to teach in Louisiana public schools.

In 1892 he returned to Texas to teach Latin at rural Mexia High School for one year, moving on from there to Navasota High School for three years and then to Temple High School until 1900. He served as principal in both localities. During this time young Kimball continued his own studies and in 1899 earned a master's degree from Baylor University in Waco. He then served as superintendent of schools in Temple from 1900 to 1902.

His career took a new turn when he moved to Waco to practice law for two years. In his words he was the "youngest member of an old law firm."[1] The firm was the court-appointed counsel for the receivership of a number of small insurance companies, so Kimball gained valuable knowledge and experience in insurance administration principles.

In 1904 he moved to Austin where he served as a law clerk in the state department of education. The next year he returned to Temple—

again as superintendent of schools. On April 12 of that year, he married Annie Lou Boggess, and in 1914 the couple moved to the growing city of Dallas, where for the next ten years he served as superintendent of schools.

Kimball was known to have a gruff manner. Though he could be harsh in his personal manner, Kimball also was known to take a sincere interest in other people, especially the teachers in his system.

During his tenure as superintendent, Kimball created and developed a number of innovations in the expanding school system.

In 1914 he introduced special classes for what society then called "mentally retarded" children, a label Kimball disregarded. The next year he lent his considerable support to the introduction of gymnasiums in Dallas schools, advancing the progressive idea that children needed physical as well as mental conditioning. In 1922 he developed a thrift program to encourage children to save money. Each Tuesday children could bring money to school and have it collected. Once a student's savings reached five dollars, the child could then open a savings account at a bank.[2]

In 1920 Baylor University awarded Kimball an honorary Doctor of Laws in commemoration of his already significant professional accomplishments.

One of his accomplishments during his tenure as superintendent in Dallas, one that would lay the foundation for his later work in group hospitalization, was setting up the Sick Benefit Fund for the school system. Several influenza epidemics made their deadly way across America and Dallas during the period. The worst, in 1918, resulted in a grim death toll of more than 500,000 nationally. Kimball, himself, came down with the flu that year.

The epidemic hit schoolteachers particularly hard financially, in part because they were not well paid and also because of harsh school system policies on extended illnesses. To Kimball the epidemic highlighted the teachers' financial problem. "The rule in those days," Kimball said, "was that if a teacher was sick enough to need a physician, enough to be in bed, she drew half pay for two weeks, and then she went off the payroll. The teacher in those circumstances . . . was in a desperate plight."[3]

In October 1921 Kimball called a meeting with leaders from the Grade Teachers Council, the High School Teachers Association and the Association of School Principals. He presented his new idea that he called the "Sick Benefit Fund," explaining that it was really a salary indemnity fund that would relieve teachers from the harsh economic impact of catastrophic illness.

Kimball had examined the absentee records of teachers in the district and announced that the average number of days lost was from 150 to

180 days per school month. He figured that if the teachers and principals paid one dollar each per month into a common fund, it would enable sick teachers to receive a payment of five dollars for each day of lost pay. To get paid, a teacher had to be sick for one week, and a physician's statement was necessary to confirm the illness.

The idea went over well. About eight hundred teachers signed up, and, at the end of the year, the Sick Benefit Fund had a surplus of more than one thousand dollars. Carrie Hughston, an elementary teacher, managed the records and accounts of the new fund.

During Kimball's ten years as superintendent, Dallas schools experienced dramatic growth. Around 1924, exhausted from his job of overseeing the burgeoning system, Kimball visited his doctor, who gave him his health options: "Slow down or break down." He replied that he wasn't going to do either. Later, he recalled thinking that "Mrs. Kimball was too young to be left a widow, and I couldn't slow down in a job like I had." His physician said, "Well, you will have to quit administrative work. I've known you twenty years, and you always do three men's work."[4]

His doctor prescribed a year-long vacation. Kimball complied with the doctor's orders by taking a year's sabbatical. While he may have quit administrative work in a technical sense, during his year off he decided to write a book. In 1924 he began writing *Our City Dallas*, subtitled "A Community Civics," written for Dallas schoolchildren. The need for the book was apparent to him. He related that "A big man in education came through Dallas one time and said, 'Kimball, I'll bet the kids of Dallas know more about the city government of ancient Athens than they do of their own city.' I had to agree with him and went to work on my book."[5]

The book was exhaustive in its detail of Dallas' history and then-current operation. It was published by the Kessler Plan Association, a group dedicated to promoting a city master plan that had earlier been presented by George Kessler. Kimball's book was published in 1927 and was used as a textbook in Dallas schools for many years.

During the time he was writing the book in the spring of 1925, he received an invitation to teach a class on educational administration at Southern Methodist University in Dallas. That summer he was named a professor of education at SMU, where he taught until 1929.

Kimball left his teaching career in 1929 when the board of trustees of Baylor University selected him as executive vice president in charge of the Dallas scientific units comprised of Baylor Hospital and the schools of medicine, nursing, pharmacy and dentistry. Kimball's primary task was to shore up the shaky financial situation of the young Dallas hospital.

Baylor was typical among the growing number of nonprofit voluntary hospitals. It was said at the time that "Methodist Hospital was in the hands of the receivers, and Baylor was just 30 days ahead of the sheriff, itself."[6] American hospitals were making a transition from being almost exclusively residential poorhouses for society's outcasts—the poor, critically ill or handicapped—to health care facilities for everyone. They had been largely places of last resort, usually financed by charity. Physicians rarely visited these almshouses, preferring to carry on their work in the more proper setting of patients' homes.

From the mid-nineteenth to the early twentieth century, a number of cultural and scientific changes hastened the birth of the modern hospital movement. Nursing became more professionalized, and health care procedures advanced—notably the discovery of anesthesia in 1846 as well as the introduction of antiseptic procedures in 1867 and X-rays in 1895. These discoveries made safer surgery possible and contributed to significantly higher rates of surgery; thus, a specialized place to perform it became necessary. Socioeconomic changes were beginning to sweep across the country as the middle class grew and people began moving to urban centers, where they were increasingly dependent upon assorted professionals, including those in health care.[7]

Financing for these growing citadels of health care technology became problematic by the 1920s. The old almshouses were financed by charity, and the early hospitals were largely supported by religious or philanthropic groups. But as the need for technology grew and the increasing sophistication of health care resulted in the need for equally sophisticated business procedures, hospitals began to shift from being places of charity to being places of business, though largely on a nonprofit basis. Hospitals began to rely more on patient payment than on charitable donations. Soon, the required price tag of improved professionalism and high technology made the simple "pay as you go" method less and less viable. Beneath all the fiscal optimism and easy credit of the 1920s, the impending hospital financing crisis would soon become an inescapable reality. In Dallas, Baylor University Hospital was caught up in the same throes.

The hospital

The hospital was founded in 1903 as Texas Baptist Memorial Sanitarium in a 14-room house. (The house that the Baptists purchased had been Good Samaritan Hospital, founded by Charles M. Rosser, M.D., in 1901.) The vision of Baylor University's board of trustees became clear: build a medical center with a national reputation. To do that, the health care complex acquired property and buildings and borrowed money to finance it.

By the 1920s the small sanitarium had been renamed Baylor Hospital and then Baylor University Hospital (after its sponsoring university). It had evolved into a sprawling (by then-standards) four hundred-bed hospital complex with a new wing for women and children as well as related schools of medicine, nursing, pharmacy and dentistry. The complex of hospital and schools came to be known as "Baylor in Dallas," with the university's board of trustees divided into two executive committees—one managing Baylor University in Waco and the other managing the "Baylor in Dallas" institutions.

Like so many other organizations of the era, the hospital and its schools were being financially seduced by easy credit, quick growth and an unrealistic optimism about the future. This false prosperity eventually brought down the American economy on the fateful "Black Thursday," October 24, 1929, with the stock market crash.

Earlier in the year, before the stock market crash, the university trustees became aware that the hospital's finances were alarmingly out of control. Their answer was to hire Kimball, a well-respected and well-connected Dallasite, and to place all of Baylor-in-Dallas' institutions under his control.

One day in 1929, Kimball was summoned to the Athletic Club in downtown Dallas by Dr. Samuel Palmer Brooks, the president of Baylor University. Brooks wanted to hire Kimball as executive vice president of Baylor University. "You run the Dallas end of it and I'll run the Waco end," Brooks offered. This commission included not only the hospital but also the affiliated health care schools.

He began his position on June 1, 1929. Just one week later, Kimball was honored at a banquet attended by 150 church and community leaders. Brooks was toastmaster for the evening. Also speaking that evening was Dr. George Truett, pastor of First Baptist Church and a man whose name would later adorn one of Baylor's future buildings. "Dr. Kimball is no novice in administrative work," Truett said that evening. "And well may we consider ourselves fortunate that we have such a man to fill this new executive post." Truett expressed the hope that Kimball could grow the Dallas units into "one of the greatest medical centers of the country." A number of other leaders expressed similar hopes.

Kimball addressed the crowd and began by declaring his reluctance to take the new job: "My new task, probably the more delicate and difficult school administrative task today in Texas, is not of my seeking or desire. It would have well contented me to have spent the rest of my working days having a modest part in the great future that lies ahead of Southern Methodist University."

Kimball then turned the topic from his interest in Dallas to broader civic concerns: how the various health care schools of the Baylor complex fared in the larger world. He suggested that Baylor University's medical college in Dallas was strategically located. He concluded his address: "Unquestionably in other ways and fields, these Baylor institutions in Dallas can be developed into valuable civic assets for our city."[8]

After the formalities of the evening came to a close, Kimball settled into the job at hand. The hospital's condition was precarious. It "was in desperate need of money and of funds and of equipment. The mattresses were worn out, and they were badly overdrawn. They owed, in current accounts and in bonds already overdue, over a million and a half in money, and that was lots of money in 1929."[9]

It was becoming clear to Kimball that a new generation of health care technology was emerging, one that required a more sophisticated funding strategy than was necessary for hospitals of previous generations. But how to do it?

The formula

As Kimball faced the situation, he thought of his earlier experience of developing the Sick Benefit Fund in the schools. In that scheme, teachers were able to pool small monthly payments that would then help pay a sick or disabled teacher's salary. Could another plan be developed that could do the same for hospitalization?

The difficulty facing Kimball was the same one that faced insurers who had considered the question of how to effectively insure one's health. It was easy to insure one's death—a person only died once, and an underwriter could look at a given population and predict with reasonable accuracy how many deaths would occur within a certain period of time. The underwriter could calculate an estimate of how much to charge (or rate) for life insurance, but it wasn't so easy to predict how often and how severely a person would get sick or injured. And with health insurance, there was the problem of adverse selection: that the person buying coverage might be doing so because of a serious illness that was contracted previously.

A few commercial health insurance companies had been started, but they had gone bankrupt. Other schemes providing some sort of financial protection against the risks of illness or accident were tried here and there but with little success. The commercial side of the industry had no accurate way to predict instances of illness or injury and so had no way to determine a rate for them.[10]

Some attempts were made to provide health care services outside the commercial insurance industry. Some lumber and logging industries had an on-site doctor to provide health care for employees. The practice was largely confined to these northwestern industries and never entered the mainstream of business or labor. In 1917 a group of textile and paper mills in North Carolina built a hospital and marketed care to employees. In 1918 a hospital in Grinell, Iowa, developed a plan similar to the one Baylor Hospital developed eleven years later, but it was not copied as was the later Baylor experiment (perhaps because the nation's hospital financing crisis had not yet become critical).

These early attempts to provide health care on a group basis were either largely unknown or produced no useful historical data on the frequency and cost of illness and accidents. Kimball quickly found that while no actuarial data existed, the old records from the Sick Benefit Fund *were* available.

That summer Kimball invited Carrie Hughston, who still managed accounts for the Sick Benefit Fund, to his office. He told her that he had studied the bills receivable of Baylor Hospital and that in the lists of bills still owed he recognized many names as being those of teachers who owed amounts up to one thousand dollars or more. Knowing that most of these teachers had no ability to afford such bills, Kimball asked to see the records of the fund so that he could study them and perhaps work out a similar plan for hospital care.

The records were familiar to him—he had designed the forms and determined what information was needed to administer the fund. Every time a teacher used the fund, a record was completed that showed which hospital was used, the length of stay, how much the hospital charged and the diagnosis—"All the information that an insurance man would want," Kimball said.

These records showed that the teachers had been spending an average of about fifteen cents per teacher a month for hospitalization. Kimball knew that with hospital services being more available, the teachers would use more. He estimated they would use twice as much as they had earlier. To make it safe, he estimated three times as much, then rounded the forty-five cents up to fifty cents and so determined his initial rate.[11]

And so the formula was invented that made group hospitalization possible. It was crude by today's sophisticated standards of actuarial science, but the idea was enough to successfully fund the early Baylor Plan.

Having created the formula, Kimball now needed to promote it. In October of that year, he went to the first school principals' meeting and told them that if they wanted a hospital plan like their Sick Benefit plan, it could be worked out. They thought well of it, and shortly thereafter Kimball sent a letter to teachers:

The plan is the outgrowth of my work some years ago with reference to the Teachers Sick Benefit Fund. Since I have been at Baylor, I have seen a number of cases of teachers, sometimes distressful, that needed the help and reinforcement of a group plan. The monthly payment is too small to be missed if one is never a beneficiary; if one is a beneficiary, it is a valuable asset in time of distress, and in many cases a blessed assistance to those in distress who are often too proud even to accept help, much less to ask for charity. For these reasons I have been studying your actuarial data and our hospital records for many weeks and submit this plan to the teachers of Dallas, confident that to none will the plan prove a burden, but on the other hand a blessing to many in the hour of pain and stress.[12]

Compared to today's comprehensive contracts, the plan was limited. It provided up to twenty-one days of care at Baylor Hospital (with a discount on regular room and board beyond that), including operating room, anesthesia and laboratory charges. In the case of an epidemic, public disaster or anything else contributing to an overcrowding of Baylor Hospital, the plan had a safeguard. If it could not provide services in these instances, it could resolve indebtedness by paying the member twice the amount of the member's premiums paid.

Enrollment went well—1,356 teachers quickly signed up, comprising about 75 percent of teachers in the district. As a result, on December 20, 1929, in the midst of one of the worst winters that Dallas and the rest of the nation had ever seen, the Group Hospitalization Plan at Baylor University Hospital in Dallas began operation. It was a date that later would be recognized as the birth of the Blue Cross movement.

2 | 1930-1944: Selling the New Idea

*"It looked like a promotional scheme and when
you went to talk to a man about it, it was
very difficult to convince him that it was
on the up-and-up."*
Lawrence Payne

On Friday, December 20, 1929, "Old King Cold" was
grabbing newspaper headlines as Dallas was in the grips of one of the
worst winter storms in its history. The evening newspaper had even reported the day before that it was warmer at the South Pole than it was in
Dallas.

The severe weather would accelerate the first use of the new group
hospitalization benefits. On December 18 or 19, a teacher in an Oak Cliff
elementary school, Alma Dickson, slipped on the icy sidewalks and hurt
her ankle. Several days later it continued to worsen, and she finally had
it examined by a physician. He discovered that a small bone was broken
just above the heel. He told her she would have to go to the hospital and
have the foot put in a cast. Dickson resisted, citing financial worries.

"Aren't you a member of this school thing they're going to try?" the
doctor countered.

"Yes," she answered, "but I don't know whether that pays the hospital bill or not. They just came around and said Dr. Kimball has another
club he wants us to work at and I paid 50 cents."[1] Dickson was admitted
to the hospital and became the first patient under the group hospitalization plan. It did, she happily discovered, really pay the hospital bill.
News of Dickson's illness and hospital care traveled quickly among the

other Dallas school teachers and became a good selling point for the Baylor Plan.

But selling the plan was not really Kimball's main interest. "My interest in the problem was primarily one of an actuarial type, having worked out a formula, having gotten an experimental group on which to provide the teachers from which I could secure actuarial data of the definite limitations, both as to origin of cost and amount of cost. Then having worked out the formula, my interest in it was primarily ended. There was a formula that would fit legally and actuarially."[2]

While Kimball may not have been a salesman, Bryce Twitty certainly was. Kimball had hired Twitty as business manager of Baylor Hospital, and Twitty soon became acting administrator, or superintendent. Twitty began work on October 15, 1929, and his attention was soon drawn to Kimball's program. Now that Kimball had developed the formula, it was time for the energetic Twitty to market the idea.

Twitty was known as a perennial optimist. Kimball claimed that he once heard Twitty say he wasn't as prepared in some things as other people, so he had to work twice as hard. And Twitty had found an idea worth working hard to sell, one he thought was "a Godsend to thousands."[3]

While the Baylor Plan's first group, the Dallas school teachers, was primarily sold through the influence and connections of Kimball, the second group was developed by Twitty. As good a salesman as Twitty was, however, it was nature that intervened to overcome the group's suspicion about the new idea.

In the summer of 1930, Twitty went to the *Dallas Morning News* office downtown to visit George Dealey, the publisher of the newspaper. Twitty described the program and said he would like to do the same thing for the newspaper's employees that was done with the Dallas school teachers.

"Well, Bryce," Dealey responded, "I don't know what it's all about but we have confidence in you and Dr. Kimball and in Baylor, and if you can enroll them, well, go at it."[4]

Twitty then went about talking to employees but found a cool reception. Many thought it sounded too good to be true. He finally enrolled one young woman, Marian Snyder Green, who was in charge of the newspaper's Biographical Department, the clipping file room known as the "morgue." She described the encounter:

> Bryce Twitty came down to the *News* and was trying to sell me on his idea for hospitalization insurance....We were fellow Baptists. I took out his prepayment plan. I couldn't lose much at the rate of 50 cents a month, and if he thought it would do any good, I was willing to try. Anything for the Baptists.
>
> It was noon, July 1, 1930, that I signed up for Bryce's plan, and I must say

I fooled myself and everyone else, for I had no idea that I would need to use it just four hours later. I had an appendicitis attack...at four o'clock, was taken to the hospital at nine o'clock, and operated on the next morning. I had stayed about a week in the hospital, and was about ready to go home, when I came down with malaria, and so I stayed over two weeks....And when I got ready to leave, my bill, which was around $150 (lots of money in those days), was completely paid. I was jubilant, of course, and Bryce didn't have any more trouble selling the plan to the employees of the *Dallas Morning News*. Bryce really put it over.[5]

The next group Twitty enrolled was the Crespi Cotton Company. There, Green's brother-in-law, Irving Honig, was instrumental in getting the program accepted by management.

With Twitty's enthusiasm pushing the concept, other familiar Dallas businesses of the era signed on: Republic National Bank, Titche-Goettinger department store, the *Daily Times Herald* newspaper and General Electric, among others. As the momentum built, Kimball and Twitty now had to start being careful not to enroll more members than Baylor Hospital could adequately handle. To ensure that Baylor Hospital could provide needed services, they set a limit of twenty-three thousand members.

In the first year of operation, a little more than one thousand members were enrolled. In that year, the Baylor experiment lost a small amount of money, but Twitty and Kimball figured that the hospital would have lost much more on bad debts had it not been for the group hospital plan.

As new groups enrolled and Baylor Hospital began to admit group hospitalization members, it became clearer that the experiment was working. Hospitals across the country were implementing similar plans. In Dallas about forty businesses prepaid their employees' hospital care through the plan, covering about four thousand members. To administer the volume of new members, Baylor hired Lawrence Payne on June 16, 1932, as director for the Group Hospitalization Department.

Twitty recruited Payne from his job at Continental Gin Company in Dallas, where Payne coordinated the group hospitalization program for Continental employees. Payne said he was destined for a career in health care because he grew up in East Dallas in the "shadow of Baylor Hospital." He met Bryce Twitty after his wife had surgery four weeks after delivering their first child.

The Paynes were able to pay for their baby's delivery but not her unexpected surgery. Twitty worked with Payne (as we assume he worked with so many others) in setting up payments through a bank to relieve Payne's hospital obligation. That wasn't the end of their hospital worries. During the first six years of the Paynes' married life, they had two babies, and his wife had four major operations. "I got in the hospital business almost in self-defense," he later joked.[6]

Public suspicion

In his years with the group hospitalization plan, the biggest obstacle Payne faced was public suspicion of the new idea. "It looked like a promotional scheme and when you went to talk to a man about it, it was very difficult to convince him that it was on the up-and-up. The hospitals...were in desperate financial condition and to sign up a group of employees to pay in on a prepaid basis to your hospital made it difficult to convince the employer that his employees' money was being safely protected. They were a little hesitant to even pay into a hospital in advance for fear that the hospital wouldn't be there to deliver the service if and when they needed it."[7]

Other hospitals in Dallas offered another challenge. Several threatened an injunction against Baylor for selling their services on a prepaid basis. One of these protestors was Dr. J. H. Groseclose, the founder and administrator of Methodist Hospital. Kimball invited Groseclose to come to Baylor and inspect for himself what the new concept was all about. Kimball said, "He was questioning the wisdom of the whole movement. I called him over the phone and invited him to come to my office and I put at his service all the information I had and I advised him knowing very well the financial status of his hospital. I advised him to go and do likewise."[8]

Groseclose did likewise but by contracting with an outside agent. He selected Clarence M. Wheeler, president of National Hospitalization System, Inc., a new company that took Kimball's idea on a commercial basis. National sold to hospitals that wanted to enter the prepaid group movement, providing them with marketing, enrollment, record keeping and collection services. Payne recalls that Wheeler would often enroll individuals at seventy-five cents a month, keeping the "extra quarter" for himself as a commission. (Quite a commission by 1930 standards!) Shortly after Methodist Hospital entered the arrangement, St. Paul Hospital in Dallas also contracted with National Hospitalization System. National had introduced Dallas' first two-hospital group plan where a subscriber could go to either hospital.

Before the decade of the 1930s ended, the Texas attorney general ruled that the National plan was really insurance and thus had to be managed under the insurance laws of the state.[9] By the late 1940s, National had faded from the scene. Though Groseclose at Methodist had contracted with National, he became an original incorporator of Group Hospital Service (which became Blue Cross of Texas) and its first president of the board in 1939. During the 1940s Methodist continued to provide hospital services through National as well as through Group Hospital Service.

The Baylor Plan also faced the ire of the Texas attorney general, perhaps because the commercial insurance companies had stirred up the situation. Twitty recalled, "The attorney general threatened to cancel the charter of Baylor if it did not cease the promotion of the plan. The fight through the Texas Legislature was bitter, but Baylor won its case. Eventually, of course, commercial insurance companies were themselves selling hospitalization insurance."[10]

Finally, the early pioneers faced the opposition of organized medicine, though hospital service plans in other parts of the country encountered stiffer opposition than did the Dallas pioneers. As news of Baylor's group hospitalization concept spread and as similar plans were set up in other parts of the country, the American Medical Association (AMA) did not welcome the new plans.

Kimball himself, in initially setting up the group hospitalization concept at Baylor Hospital, had very carefully drawn the idea to avoid getting between the physician in private practice and the patient. "I had never conferred with the Dallas doctors as to this plan," he said. "I carefully drew the plan so it would not impinge or infringe in any way on a doctor's relationship between himself and his patient."[11] This would set the tone for the industry's relationship with physicians for another fifty years.

Kimball's reluctance to get in the way of the patient-physician relationship was a reflection of how, by the end of the first quarter of the twentieth century, medical practice had consolidated itself as an organized profession. Such had not always been the case.

In the nineteenth century, medical practice in the United States had few professional education standards and was divided into competing healing sects. By the end of that century, the medical profession was comprised mostly of individuals from three competing schools of thought: the "eclectics," who used herbal medicine along with the conventional remedies of the era; the "homeopaths," who tried to cure disease by giving drugs that produced the same symptoms in an attempt to boost the body's natural immune system; and the "regulars," also called allopaths, who used the scientific approach to relieve symptoms and cure illness by drugs and surgery.

By the early part of the twentieth century, physicians had primarily adopted the scientific approach. This was due in part to the increasingly scientific nature of a culture that was becoming more urbanized and specialized and in part because the "regulars" actually cured more illnesses than the others.

Once physicians had a common methodology and language, they consolidated their strength and autonomy as a profession by improving the quality of medical education, advancing the state of medical technology and working to enhance their own professionalism.[12]

In the pre-World War I days, it looked as if the nation's physicians would support a nationalized health care program. Some early leaders of the AMA initially supported legislation for a nationalized system, but as the idea went forward, first business, then organized medicine, opposed it. Also, the nation's entry into World War I against Germany turned public opinion against nationalized health insurance even more, since Germany had established the first national system of compulsory sickness insurance in 1883.

By the time Baylor's group hospitalization plan was created, organized medicine did not support any form of "compulsory insurance," as they termed it. On the contrary in Dallas, where the group hospitalization concept was born, doctors were more neutral, if not somewhat open to the idea. This was likely due to Kimball's rubbing elbows with Edward H. Cary, M.D., a prominent ophthalmologist with a reputation for being outspoken.

Cary is credited with vastly improving medical education in Dallas. As a young man he was drawn to study ophthalmology after suffering severe eye difficulties himself as a child. He served without pay as the first dean of the Baylor College of Medicine from the school's beginning in 1902 until 1921. He was later credited with starting Southwestern Medical College in Dallas after Baylor's medical school moved to Houston. He became president of the AMA in 1932 and a staunch opponent of nationalized health insurance as the head of the National Physicians Committee during the post-World War II years. But Cary didn't oppose the Baylor Plan, and his influence undoubtedly kept local physician resistance to the new idea at a minimum. Kimball credited this to some degree to his association with Cary in a dinner club where the two were acquainted and apparently had come to respect each other. Cary said he was once asked about the "ethics" of the new hospitalization plan, and he responded, "I don't know anything about the plan. But if Kimball drew it, it's ethical all right. I know Kimball."[13]

While later Cary aggressively fought any form of compulsory or socialized medicine, in time he championed the voluntary prepaid hospitalization movement and became president of the board of Blue Cross and Blue Shield of Texas, serving until his death in 1953 at age 81.

Lawrence Payne recalled that the Dallas doctors recognized the potential benefit of better hospitalization for more people. "The doctors realized that even though it may not be 'according to Hoyle,' they knew that it was doing something for their patient and in the final analysis was doing something for them. They were getting the hospital bill out of the way and it made it easier for a doctor to collect his own bill. So, when you talk about the doctors' attitude, the ones who actually experienced it seemed to be pretty well wholeheartedly for it. I think the opposition came primarily from those who had not had the opportunity to experience this movement."[14]

Despite these challenges, the Baylor group hospitalization concept continued to spread slowly to more businesses across Dallas. One boost to sales came when Kimball agreed to allow a family contract, covering not only the employee but also the employee's family as well.

Kimball was initially reluctant to introduce coverage for spouses and children, fearing that it would adversely affect the rate. He thought that malingering could become a problem. While an employee had an incentive to stay out of the hospital and at work, it was reasoned that the spouse (the wife in most cases) would not have that incentive and might use hospitalization as a "rest cure."

However, in 1933 Baylor offered the family contract at a rate of one dollar per month, due mainly to public demand. Payne recalled:

> I kept having difficulty with the employee – the man, for instance, who said, "I don't need this for myself but I do need it for my family, my wife and children." Of course, I knew that because I was having the same experience. And we went back and talked to Mr. Twitty and Dr. Kimball in a very pleading sort of way many times and expressed my experiences with these groups, showed them how much more quickly we could get them enrolled and how much more good we could do if we could put in the family plan. And along in 1933…we worked out a family plan whereby the family would…get the same benefits that the employee got, except they would pay half of their room rent regardless of what room they went into.[15]

The one dollar per month rate for the family plan and the fifty cents per month rate for the employee-only were undoubtedly bargains, even in that day. The employee-only rate remained at fifty cents per month until 1934. Data collected showed that some groups were using more services, and some were using less, so the plan shifted to pricing its services through "experience rating," based on the actual health experience of the group.

Depending on past experience, groups were charged from fifty cents to seventy-five cents per member each month, but this rate was set once the group was enrolled. Even if the group's experience exceeded the premium level, it was not charged more. "We just watched it," Payne recalled. At one point, however, Payne said they had to move the department stores and school teachers above seventy-five cents. (This may have been the world's first health insurance rate increase.)

As Payne continued to market the program, he became more aware of the limitations of a single hospital plan. In emergencies, people needed to go to the closest hospital, not necessarily the one where they had pre-paid care. In addition, members had to be careful to select only those physicians who had admitting privileges at Baylor. Payne recalled one case in which an injured woman was hospitalized seventy-five miles out-side of Dallas. Although her entire family was covered in the Baylor pro-gram, she was too seriously injured to be moved to Baylor and so her hospitalization was not covered.

While Dallas' early experiment in group hospitalization never got beyond one hospital, such was not true elsewhere as events in the nation fueled the evolution of the group hospitalization concept.

The concept spreads

It didn't take long for the nation's hospitals to notice the success of the Baylor experiment in Dallas. In 1930 Kimball attended the American Hospital Association (AHA) convention in New Orleans. He was in a meeting when the subject of prepaid hospitalization was mentioned. Kimball was called upon to tell the group about the Dallas prepayment plan. He told his story, and word spread throughout the AHA convention about the apparent success of the Baylor experiment.

Across the nation, hospitals took notice of what was happening in Dallas, and opinions varied greatly about the experiment. Twitty said that some hospital officials supported the concept, seeing it as a way to keep their hospitals open during the difficult depression years. Others were opposed, saying it was unethical and unsound. The arguments among members of AHA were heated, Twitty said, and "it seemed that no one was on the fence. Everybody was violently for or violently opposed to it."[16]

One person who heard about what was going on in Dallas was Frank Van Dyk, executive secretary of the Essex County Hospital Council in New Jersey. Van Dyk had grappled with the same economic issues facing hospitals as had Kimball and a score of other people across the nation. His job was to collect bad debts from former patients of the seventeen hospitals in the council. He worked out payment arrangements with many of these patients, so that patients gradually paid their debts at the rate of one or two dollars per week or per month.

An idea emerged: If they could do that *after* the fact, they could do it *before* they were burdened and pay in advance. Van Dyk said that thought led to another thought: "How wonderful it would be to remove the cashier's department from a hospital and permit people to go to a hospital as a patient rather than as a customer."[17] Kimball's plan seemed to fit his own emerging sense of how to better finance hospital care, so he decided to come to Dallas and see for himself how the program was working out.

In 1932 he arrived in Dallas and went first to the offices of National Hospitalization System, thinking that this was the group hospitalization plan he had heard about. He then learned it was not. "My reaction was wholly adverse to that idea because hospitals were voluntary nonprofit institutions. I felt that making profit out of this kind of an arrangement was unwarranted and unjustified and against public interest."[18]

He went immediately to Baylor University Hospital. There he found Twitty and got the details of how the "real" Baylor Plan was developed and how well it was working. Twitty then suggested he talk to Cary, who likewise told Van Dyk what he knew about the development of the plan. Cary then referred him to other members of the Dallas County Medical Society, of which Cary was then president.

Van Dyk also conferred with some of the plan's enrolled groups, including the Titche-Goettinger department store, where he spoke with the personnel manager and some employees who were members of the Baylor Plan. "I found general satisfaction with the plan as long as they could go to the Baylor University Hospital and their doctors practiced there. I found no adverse comment about the movement or the plan itself, other than the fact that it seemed quite obvious that the idea was an excellent one but that it ought to be on a community-wide basis. . . . Unless there was an established general community-wide plan, there would be interference with their free choice of physician and free choice of hospital."[19]

Van Dyk returned to New Jersey and discussed the idea of a community-wide plan with the board of directors of the Essex County Hospital Council. It became operational on January 1, 1933, and was the nation's first nonprofit multi-hospital plan. (In July 1932 a multi-hospital plan was established in Sacramento, California, as a for-profit venture.) Van Dyk's program became a model for such community-wide plans, and similar programs were begun elsewhere.

One such group hospital plan, an eight-hospital plan in St. Paul, Minnesota, hired an enterprising young man to be its manager. E. A. van Steenwyk had worked in a number of fields, including publishing, and so he understood the need to market the group hospitalization idea. He needed a symbol or a mark that would distinguish his plan and quickly went about developing one.

He first created a cartoon figure, Sally the Student Nurse. Van Steenwyk recalled, "Sally did not have the kind of long-term currency that you needed. You needed something that didn't change over a long period of time. We used for Sally a blue and white uniform. That blue and white was the basis for the idea of the blue cross. The hospital, of course, had always used a cross, so that was a natural use of a cross."[20]

Van Steenwyk commissioned a poster by distinguished artist Joseph Bender in a sleek, airbrushed, art deco style, showing a nurse's arm cradling a wounded head. On the nurse's sleeve was a blue cross. The image was what the movement needed. Across the nation, most of the hospital service associations (as they were then called) began to identify themselves with this mark.

Plans were burgeoning across the nation, and the AHA began to see the need for some sort of national structure and standards for the various plans. An organization that was instrumental in lending support to the AHA to develop standards was the Julius Rosenwald Fund in Chicago. The fund employed Rufus Rorem, a professor of accounting at the University of Chicago, and lent his services to the AHA to study the emerging prepaid hospital movement and the experience of these divergent plans.

In 1936 the Rosenwald Fund offered Rorem's services and $100,000 to the AHA, so that Rorem could continue his work. The AHA accepted and created the Committee on Hospital Service, and Rorem himself was named an associate director of the AHA. This committee evolved into the Blue Cross Commission.

In 1937 Rorem called the first national meeting of prepaid hospital plan executives in Chicago in order to share experiences and ideas. At the meeting the AHA unveiled fourteen membership standards that would qualify plans to display the official Blue Cross logo. By now, the cross logo had been adorned with the official seal of the AHA at its center.

By the following year when the standards went into effect, thirty-eight Plans were in place with more than a million members collectively. The Blue Cross concept was maturing to national standing.[21]

The end of the Baylor Plan

As Blue Cross was becoming a well-known national entity with a bright future, the Baylor Plan in Dallas was coming to the end of its short but historic course. By 1934 the Baylor Plan reached its saturation point of twenty-three thousand members.

The last group sold was Cabell's Milk and Ice Cream Company, when Ben and Earl Cabell gave their employees the group hospitalization plan for one year as a Christmas present. The Baylor Plan stopped taking groups on December 24, 1934. The plan marketed itself for only the first five of its fifteen years of existence. For the next ten years, the plan serviced the groups it had and welcomed new employees of existing groups but did not open its membership to more businesses.

Lawrence Payne, who had been director of the Group Hospitalization Department at Baylor, became assistant administrator of the hospital but left in 1938 to be an administrator for a Waco hospital. He returned to Baylor Hospital in 1943 as administrator and set to work giving all Baylor Plan members the opportunity to transfer to Blue Cross of Texas.

By December 31, 1944, the Baylor Plan ceased operation. The experiment had started a revolution in a most simple way and in an era when health care and health care financing were still in their infancy. The challenge facing Kimball and the other pioneers in those years had been just a matter of paying for health care "a nickel at a time." As Payne said:

> Early studies showed that the nation spent practically the same amount on chewing gum during those three years prior to 1929 as they did for hospital bills and spent three times the amount on tobacco as they did for hospital bills. Dr. Kimball and Bryce Twitty frequently said that "all we are trying to do is put the hospital bill on a chewing gum basis and let you pay for it, a nickel at a time...then you won't call us highway robbers."

> It was also determined that one out of fourteen persons went to the hospital each year during those years. That meant that each one of us would average once in fourteen years. We could go to the grocery store and buy a loaf of bread in those days for a dime a loaf or less and nobody complained about it because we paid for it day by day. But if we had to buy a fourteen-year demand of bread all at one time, it would have cost more than $500. This would have placed bread out of reach of most people in those days the same as hospital services were out of their reach. These were the things that caused Dr. Kimball to want to develop a plan that most people could reach. He frequently said that it was not the high cost of hospital bills that creates such a burden, but the lack of distribution of that cost over a period of years.[22]

This "nickel-at-a-time" formula proved inadequate in later years as health care technology became more sophisticated and health care financing more problematic. However, it was enough to start a revolution that would benefit millions of people across the nation.

By the time the Baylor Plan had run its course, the revolution had come full circle and returned to Texas as a small group of hospital leaders struggled to build a hospitalization plan across the great expanse of the Lone Star State.

Part Two

The Story of Blue Cross and Blue Shield of Texas

3 | 1939-1941: Shaky Beginnings

*"I intend to put this over in a great way and
we will have one of the finest plans in America here
in Texas and it will be a blessing to humanity for
many years to come."*
Bryce Twitty

A decade had passed since the Baylor Plan was founded, and in that period the group hospitalization concept spread quickly across the nation. This was in no small part because of the Depression that was wreaking havoc on all sectors of American life, including health care. The state medical journal reported, "Many violent storms are passing over the medical profession of Texas and the nation. The trend of economic affairs, accentuated by the continued economic depression, has precipitated a feeling of unrest, fraught with serious possibilities."[1]

One of those serious possibilities was nationalized health care. A mandated national health care program was originally in President Roosevelt's Social Security Act but was dropped at the eleventh hour because it was feared that its controversy would endanger the overall act from passing. Neither the hospital nor the medical profession supported a national health care plan. "The medical profession is opposed to the socialization of medicine," proclaimed an editorial in the same issue of the state medical magazine, "rather because of the anticipated ill effects upon the dependent public, than upon the welfare of its own members, although its effect upon the profession of medicine would be most shameful and baneful. It is felt that the effect of socializing medicine would be to destroy the personal relationship of the physician to his patient, which is, after all, the basic and most important principle involved in practice."[2]

Among hospital professionals and a growing number of physicians, the group hospitalization movement was seen as a remedy to creeping federal bureaucracy. Certainly, it was proving itself as a practical remedy to the continued economic pressures facing both hospitals and patients.

The group hospitalization plan at Baylor Hospital had started a movement of similar programs at hospitals around the country. The Texas State Hospital Association (TSHA—later in the decade to be known simply as the Texas Hospital Association) took an early interest in the Baylor Plan. At the 1931 annual meeting of TSHA at John Sealy Hospital in Galveston, Kimball presented the principles of the Baylor group hospitalization plan. He said that since the program had begun, Baylor Hospital had been operating at between 80 and 85 percent of its bed capacity—certainly a statistic that grabbed the attention of cash-flow starved hospital administrators at the start of the Depression.

As the decade progressed, officials of TSHA became more interested in having a community-wide hospital plan in Texas. Already, various individual hospital plans were in existence around the state. Baylor, Methodist and St. Paul hospitals in Dallas all had plans competing with each other. Two major Fort Worth hospitals and one in San Antonio had plans as well.

Physicians likewise began to take note of the emerging movement. In December 1934, some Dallas physicians met in the home of Dr. C. M. Rosser to discuss prepayment plans. They decided that any local plan should be designed to be of benefit only to the person of moderate means, amounts charged should be reasonable and fees paid in line with actual fees. Especially, they thought, patients should have the choice of "reputable physicians."[3]

On January 7, 1939, the board of trustees of the (now named) Texas Hospital Association (THA) were meeting and their attorney, Phil Overton, was charged with pursuing legislation that would enable a non-profit group hospitalization company in Texas to be formed. Such an act was needed in Texas, as in most states, because existing insurance laws or legislation provided only for insurance company-type operations and not hospital service plans. In Texas, as elsewhere, plans would never have been started had they been considered mere insurance companies; they could not possibly have assembled the capital or adequately set reserves.

In April THA members met in their annual assembly at the Hotel Texas in Fort Worth and heard John Mannix of Detroit talk about "the future of voluntary hospitals." Mannix, a gifted young hospital administrator, hailed from Cleveland, Ohio, where he helped organize that city's prepayment plan. By 1939 he was executive director of the Michigan Society for Group Hospitalization. Later, he became a national leader in the Blue Cross and Blue Shield System, calling (unsuccessfully) for the consolidation of the independent plans into a single, national organization. Twitty, who by this time had become legislative chairman of THA, had asked Mannix to come to Texas, most likely as an incentive to spur events along and to get the enabling act passed. In addition to addressing THA, Mannix spent three days in a series of meetings with members of both houses of the Texas Legislature.

Mannix told the assembly that the voluntary prepayment movement would safeguard hospitals from eventual control by the federal government and that if voluntary hospitals were to survive, some method of financing must be developed. He asserted that the group hospitalization concept was that method of financing. "These hospital plans must be made available to everyone in the United States if the voluntary institutions are to survive. These plans not only assume hospitalization but they lift a tax burden from the people by supporting the voluntary hospitals and eliminating the need for government support."[4]

At the board meeting during the assembly, members appointed the incorporators of the new group hospitalization company, to be comprised of THA leaders who would meet the following month to incorporate the new organization, assuming passage of the new bill.

The bill passed both houses of the Texas Legislature during the forty-sixth legislative session, and the governor signed it into law. It provided for the establishment of non-profit organizations for the purpose of "furnishing group hospital service." It did the following:

- Gave any such organization the authority to contract with hospitals to furnish hospital services to subscribers;
- Prohibited contracting for medical services;
- Mandated that no more than 15 percent of "dues" could be used for administration expense;
- Limited the salary of any employee to six thousand dollars per year (with all salaries to be approved by the Board of Insurance Commissioners);
- Provided that a majority of the board of directors be directors, superintendents or trustees of hospitals that contract or may contract with the organization; and
- Provided for supervision by the Insurance Commission.

The bill only authorized the *forming* of such non-profit group hospitalization ventures; it did not actually create any organizations. That task—and it was to be a difficult one—was the challenge of THA leaders as they created Group Hospital Service, Inc. (GHS).[5]

The incorporation

GHS was the nation's fifty-ninth group hospital plan organized. The other fifty-eight plans were in twenty-four states, with most of the plans covering local areas within states.[6] In later years almost all of these regional plans were consolidated into statewide organizations and sometimes multi-state operations.

All the incorporators were THA leaders. The president of THA that year was Dr. J. H. Groseclose who had set up a group plan at Methodist Hospital in Dallas to compete with the Baylor Plan. Groseclose's early career was as a minister in the Methodist church. He held pastorates in Tennessee and in Texas at Laredo, San Antonio, Uvalde, Beeville and Temple, and was presiding elder of the San Antonio and Beeville districts. In 1920 he was awarded an honorary doctor of divinity degree from Emory and Henry College in Emory, Virginia, and the next year the North Texas Conference of the Methodist church appointed him superintendent of the proposed Methodist Hospital in Dallas. He supervised construction and operation of that hospital and remained as superintendent until his death in 1943. He was on the THA board of trustees in 1937-38 and was elected president in 1939. In 1942 he was named as a trustee of the American Hospital Association (AHA).

The enabling legislation thus secured, Groseclose called a meeting of the incorporators at the Driskill Hotel in Austin on May 23, 1939, at 10 a.m. Assembled in the room with Groseclose were:

- Ara Davis, Superintendent of Scott and White Hospital in Temple and THA's President Elect;
- C. E. Hunt, Superintendent of Lubbock Sanitarium and Clinic and a member of THA's Government Relations Council;
- L. N. Markham, M.D., Superintendent of Markham-McRee Hospital in Longview and THA's Vice President;
- Martha Roberson, Superintendent of Medical and Surgical Memorial Hospital in San Antonio and a THA trustee;
- Josie M. Roberts, Superintendent of Methodist Hospital in Houston and a THA trustee.
- Margaret Hales Rose, Superintendent of Wichita General Hospital, Wichita Falls, and THA's second vice president, was the only incorporator not in attendance as she was out of state.

Also in the room were Bryce Twitty, still superintendent of Baylor Hospital; Phil Overton, who had husbanded the enabling legislation into law; notary public Jane Glass Laney; and Madelyne Sturdavant, Groseclose's secretary, who served as secretary of the meeting. The group discussed the charter to be prepared, agreed upon the name of Group Hospital Service, Inc., and Dallas as its home office.

The first item of business was to elect officers. Groseclose was elected president, Markham, vice president, and Roberts, secretary-treasurer. Markham nominated Twitty as the organization's administrator. Groseclose asked him if he would accept the position with the understanding that THA was no longer financially responsible to the group and that all expenses of the company, including Twitty's salary, would be paid when funds were available. Twitty agreed and added that he needed authority to select personnel for the local offices throughout the state without having to go back to the board. The board agreed. Twitty would leave Baylor Hospital saying he had been granted an indefinite leave of absence as superintendent and devote his full energies to the new corporation. The board offered Overton the position of counselor for the corporation and told him that he would be paid when funds were available. Twitty presented two membership contracts he had drafted. The board made various suggestions, and Twitty was asked to present revised contracts at the next meeting. The meeting adjourned at 4:15 p.m.

On Saturday, June 10, the group assembled again, this time in Dallas at the Baker Hotel. The meeting spanned two days, through Sunday afternoon, since so many details had to be worked out.

The subscriber's certificate or contract was approved. It provided for:

- Either private room or ward accommodations (for which the hospital was paid $5 per day and $3.50 per day, respectively);
- Maternity care after twelve months;
- The inclusion of dependents at one-half the room allowance but otherwise the same benefits;
- Choice of hospital;
- Cancellation by either party on thirty days written notice;
- Payment *to* the hospital for benefits given *to* the subscriber (the most important feature of the contract).

Monthly rates were set: Seventy-five cents for employed men, eighty-five cents for employed women, sixty-five cents for adult dependents and twenty cents for minor dependents.

The contract with hospitals was developed: The hospital was prohibited from collecting from the patient any charges covered by the subscriber contract, although the hospital could collect for services rendered but not included in the subscriber contract. GHS agreed to pay the hospital its charges for the subscriber benefits the patient used.

Proposed bylaws were presented and adopted. The board adopted Twitty's salary at six thousand dollars (the limit, according to the enabling act). They also adopted a temporary budget of six thousand dollars for the first three months. Twitty was charged with going to Austin to present the Plan of Operation to the insurance commissioner.

The commissioner allowed GHS to set up its headquarters in Dallas. Twitty reported that Nathan Adams, president of the First National Bank of Dallas and chairman of a special committee formed by the Dallas Chamber of Commerce, had announced to him that twenty-five thousand dollars had been raised from various Dallas businesses to start the new hospitalization organization. It was a loan, not a gift, to be repaid out of the 15 percent allowed for administrative expense.

Funding the new company

The initial organizing done, the real work began. Twitty went to work raising funds, hiring staff, leasing offices around the state, marketing the plan, enrolling subscribers and talking up the new company wherever he went.

Funding the company was his initial challenge. In other areas of the country, plans had been started from grants, foundations, community funds, hospitals or hospital associations. Texas had no local hospital councils and few (if any) other groups with funding for community endeavors. Money had to be raised in an entrepreneurial fashion by telling people of the high-mindedness and public spirit of the new company and asking for a loan, if not a donation. Given the huge geographic territory of the state, this would not be an easy task.

The loan of twenty-five thousand dollars came only after many letters, phone calls and visits to business leaders of Dallas. Twitty's correspondence from the era tells the tale of his vast challenge as well as of his promoter personality as he painted the utopian picture of a company that would aid millions of Texans. To the president of a Dallas bank:

> A conservative estimate is that within the course of two or three years that probably a million people in Texas will be covered on this plan. It is a civic non-profit hospitalization plan whereas we are to sell protection to the masses of people at a low rate....You can readily see that the plan will have an enormous organization. The income will run from two to three million dollars annually, and will have an office personnel ultimately of three hundred people....In order to get started the directors feel that we should have at least $25,000....I wish you would ask the Clearing House Association to appropriate at once as much money as they can possibly do—not less than $1,000.[7]

Twitty was not above pitting one community against another to raise money. To Markham of Longview he wrote:

> ...(W)e do not have a penny in the drawer now and we will have to run a

month or two before we have any to amount to anything. It is imperative, therefore, that we have some money. Tell these men whom you call upon that this is a civic non-profit organization and one of the greatest social movements for the betterment of a social problem among the people that we have had in several decades....Won't you do this this week and see if you cannot let us have from your fine town at least $1,000. Hunt is raising $1,000 at Lubbock. I know that you should be able to raise $5,000 in Longview if $1,000 can be raised at Lubbock.[8]

If it would help raise money, he was not afraid to suggest that the home office should be in another city. To Groseclose in Dallas he wrote:

If Dallas doesn't want to raise the $25,000, I already have the assurance that Houston will and you know that if Amon Carter knows that $25,000 would put the headquarters in Fort Worth he would raise this amount of money overnight.[9]

He also was not afraid to ask others to become volunteer fundraisers for the new company, making it sound as if it were a duty to humanity. To Hunt in Lubbock:

We feel that you can raise from $1,000 to $5,000 in Lubbock without any trouble....Won't you, therefore, please immediately ask these people to share in this work with us? It is a civic matter. The greatest gift on earth you give to any friend is to help him help himself, and not to give him charity. That is exactly what group hospital service does. It helps them to help each other without receiving charity. I wish you would see about this at any early date and let us have the money, making it payable to Group Hospital Service, Inc.[10]

Setting up a statewide company in a territory as big as Texas would require an automobile, of course. He sent the same letter to officials of the local Ford, Dodge, Oldsmobile and Buick dealerships in Dallas:

As you know, Baylor originated group hospitalization ten years ago. We have given nearly a million dollars worth of service on the plan....Therefore, I am writing this letter to present for your consideration a request for the gift of two automobiles to the Group Hospital Service of Texas, Inc....There is necessarily quite an expense involved in organizing a company with the scope of this organization, particularly in the vast state of Texas, so it is necessary to call upon public-spirited people and large employers of labor for aid in underwriting this expense. We expect to use quite a number of cars for our sales people in two years time, and will most certainly feel obligated to make this a Ford (or Oldsmobile, or Buick, or Dodge) account if given this start by your company.[11]

The appeals were unsuccessful, although Twitty was able to purchase a Dodge at factory cost.

While twenty-five thousand dollars was needed to start the Dallas headquarters, money was also raised from communities around the state. Like the twenty-five thousand dollars in Dallas, most of the money from area communities were loans, not donations. While Wichita Falls, Amarillo, San Benito, Longview, Tyler, Lubbock, San Antonio and Houston gave loans, San Angelo and Waco gave donations. Most, though not all, of the funds came from hospitals. A total of a little more than six thousand dollars was raised from these communities. These loans and gifts from smaller cities proved problematic—communities that gave money were expecting to see a local office opened in their city, and Twitty was ready to promise such an office if it would result in more funds.

Regardless of Twitty's hints of other cities wanting the headquarters of GHS, there is no other indication that any city besides Dallas was ever seriously considered. After all, Dallas was recognized already as the birthplace of group hospitalization, and it was only right and logical, so it seemed to the early leaders, that GHS would find its genesis in Dallas. The first office was set to open on July 10, 1939, in a two-room suite, No. 204, in the majestic Medical Arts Building in downtown Dallas.

Just before the company actually began operation, civic leaders of Dallas honored Twitty with a dinner on July 6. A decade earlier, Dallas dignitaries had hosted a gala honoring Kimball, acknowledging their faith in his ability to help Baylor Hospital. Now, a dinner was to launch the new statewide hospitalization plan by honoring its first administrator, the well-known Twitty. The Dallas County Medical Society, Baylor Hospital and the Rotary Club sponsored the appreciation dinner at the Dallas Athletic Club. Before the speeches, those gathered witnessed the message "Good Luck Bryce" molded in ice letters about three feet square.

Groseclose and Cary and other representatives of the sponsoring organizations gave speeches praising Twitty. Then it was the honoree's turn to talk. He spoke idealistically of the potential of the organization:

> To benefit by the plan will not be a burden on any person who has a permanent income. The tenant farmer can sell milk and butter to pay the premium to protect himself and his family. The ribbon counter clerk can pay the small assessment without feeling the burden. This service fills the gap between what it costs the hospital to serve patients in case of illness and what the patient can pay when in need of this service. The public is not to view this plan with that of insurance, but to remember that it is a service corporation originated by hospital people to render hospital service to the public at actual cost. It is a nonprofit corporation for service only....It is not charity but a method whereby a person may budget his hospital bill. The plan makes it possible for the person who would otherwise have to have charity to pay his way and retain his self respect.[12]

With the formalities out of the way, it was time to get down to the details of business. The July 9 board meeting convened in Galveston in conjunction with the THA board of trustees meeting. It was a short meeting, letting out at noon, but already the details of doing business were pressing for attention. What percentage of a group's employees should be required to enroll? The board voted two-thirds of eligible employees. Should the company contract with tax-supported hospitals? The board voted that those tax-supported hospitals that also accepted private-pay patients could be issued contracts but only with board approval. Where should branch offices be? Several communities around the state were requesting (and in some cases, pressuring for) offices. The board decided not to act on this yet but to tell the communities that their request would be considered later. A proposed budget was submitted, amounting to $35,000, with $16,500 of that salaries for Twitty ($6,000), four salesmen ($1,200 each), a controller ($2,400) and three support staff ($3,300).

Groseclose sent out a letter to THA-member hospitals, explaining the new corporation and alerting them that Twitty would be sending them a contract for their review. Contracts began coming in, and an alliance of hospitals across the state began forming.

Someone was needed to market the plan and, until salesmen were hired, the directors themselves sometimes worked to enroll groups, usually orchestrated by Twitty. Roberson in San Antonio wrote Twitty: "I have an inquiry today for hospitalization from the Magnolia Oil Company of Luling and the Gunter Hotel of this city. I am going to make a personal appointment with the Chairman of the Gunter Hotel Group, and I am writing to the Luling people to get in touch with you."[13]

To which Twitty responded:

> Just as soon as we get the policies out, let me send them to you, and will you contact the Magnolia people....We want payroll deduction. If you will forward them the policy and write it yourself, you will save us that much overhead. However, if you feel it necessary I shall be happy indeed to make a special trip there for it. I would caution you to go easy on the Gunter Hotel. Our experience with hotels has been pretty bad. The labor turnover is mighty fast....However we are making a profit on the Adolphus at this time. The only way you can be profitable on the hotel is to take the whole group and not let just a few, who feel the need of operation, take it out. If you can sign these up it will certainly be a help, and God knows we need the help.

As usual, he gave Roberson a pep talk at the close of the letter:

> Everybody seems to think this is the brightest idea that has come through in the past ten years. Our papers say that it is a wonderful blessing to humanity

and a Godsend to the hospitals....Some think I am nuts for leaving Baylor, a cinch, and go into this speculative work. But I know that if I make a success of this the Board of Directors will pay me well. This job ought to pay $9,000 a year as soon as the volume will justify. I know our directors will be happy to pay it when that time comes. You will be interested to know that our Trustees refused to accept my resignation and told me to take a leave of absence for such time as I need....Of course, I never intend to return because I intend to put this thing over in a great way and we will have one of the finest plans in America here in Texas and it will be a blessing to humanity for many years to come.[14]

Twitty and several directors thought area offices should be set up at once so the company could establish itself across the state quickly, both to fend off any government-imposed plan and to compete with commercial companies that were already legion in the state. He required communities to raise enough funds for three months of operating expense before he would consider putting in an office. In August he recommended that offices be opened in cities that had provided funds: Tyler, Longview, Amarillo, Waco, San Benito, Houston and Dallas. He also suggested that offices be opened in San Angelo, Lubbock, El Paso, San Antonio and Wichita Falls, as soon as they qualified by providing enough funds. A few board members, including Groseclose himself, suggested slowing down the process of opening new offices, getting each established before taking on too many. Roberson was pushing for an office in San Antonio, even ahead of the required funding. She suggested to Twitty that she might like to retire from hospital work and take over the San Antonio office, which she eventually did within the next year, stepping down from the board.

Twitty thought that not only *should* the company expand quickly but also that it *would* if only enough effort were put forth. He foresaw the day when virtually every Texan would be covered by GHS. He was convinced that day would come if only he and the others would push enough and get people's attention along with their enrollment cards. In a letter to Robert Jolly, administrator of Memorial Hospital in Houston, he wrote once again of his vision:

In Texas, we are running ten plans in one, and from the beginning it was my idea that each plan have its own Advisory Board. That is why we have deposited the money there in Houston. The Dallas office is in reality the consolidating or coordinating office, which is far better than having ten different independent plans in Texas. All of the plans are going to go statewide, and all they have started this year have begun on statewide basis, because you cannot take some little nook and corner of the state and sell the plan, because of the mobility of the people in moving as well as traveling. Texas being an oil state, large groups of families move from one section to the other, according to oil production.[15]

When he wasn't writing letters to health care leaders across the state, Twitty was traveling around the state, trying to establish an office here, drum up another account there, hiring staff, trying in general to launch the statewide entity of GHS.

The next board meeting was scheduled for August 29 at the Baker Hotel in Dallas. Jolly of Houston and Lucius R. Wilson, M.D., of John Sealy Hospital in Galveston were elected to the board. Then, Groseclose abruptly announced his resignation, citing his responsibilities as superintendent of Methodist Hospital in Dallas and president of THA. Health was really the predominant factor, for he had a serious heart condition, and the duties of starting a new corporation were proving burdensome on his frail health. He said, however, that he wished to remain on the board, but not as president. Later in the day, the board named Wilson as the second president and chairman of the board of GHS. Both Wilson and Jolly had engaged Groseclose in critical correspondence and perhaps it became the board's perception that Wilson would make a good successor.

Wilson was a charter member and first president of TSHA. He also was a charter member of the American College of Hospital Administrators and its president in 1934.

At the same meeting, the board added two of Dallas' most prominent citizens. Cary, a physician of national stature because of his AMA leadership and of his campaign against nationalized health care, began what was to be an exemplary tenure of leadership. George B. Dealey, owner and publisher of the *Dallas Morning News* and WFAA radio, added another very recognizable Dallas name to the board. These appointments were effective October 1.

The board approved paying salesmen a commission—fifty cents per certificate and five cents per mile for expenses when driving outside their immediate town. Later, the commission proved troublesome because it encouraged enrollment regardless of the health condition of the applicant, and it violated a principle of the AHA—that selling the prepayment plans should be on a non-commission basis.

Another question was over which hospitals were eligible to be GHS Member Hospitals. Should hospitals be "listed" by the Texas Hospital Association (which is what the original subscriber contract said) or be actual members of THA? Should hospitals be approved by the AMA (which several doctors on the board thought ought to be required), and, if so, what about hospitals that had applied for AMA approval but had not yet been accepted? In typical fashion Jolly wrote Wilson (copying the other board members) and asked him the hard questions. In a letter to Wilson, Twitty answered Jolly's question about hospital eligibility and then, showing frustration over what he considered to be a picky question, replied pointedly (with a copy sent to each board member):

> It is hard to be patient with small things like this when we are doing our best, working ten and fifteen hours a day trying to make this plan a success, in competition with cut-throat commercial companies. We are doing our best to keep these hospitals from being taken over by the federal government, which is definitely so unless Group Hospital Service, Inc. is successful....What hospital people need to be doing instead of trying to find some fault is to get behind this with every ounce of strength they have and help push it over. We are working with practically no capital, and in spite of the high-pressure salesmanship, unlimited advertising expenditures and untrue statements made by commercial companies, we are making rapid success.[16]

Wilson responded sharply, stating that he saw no reason why he could not raise "any question at any time" about the operation of the company. He even threatened to resign as president if other situations as this developed, saying "I definitely did not want to be president of the organization and still do not want to be president of it."[17] (Indeed, his tenure as president was short. Groseclose was re-elected president at the February 21, 1940, meeting.)

Growing concern

Administering the details of the new company became more and more complex for the directors. Unfortunately, it was becoming apparent that Twitty did not have a firm grasp of the details or much control on the administration of either the area offices or the central office. The task facing Twitty was probably more than any one person could be expected to handle, especially with such a meager budget in such a large geographic area.

Some of the directors began to get uncomfortable. Groseclose at first suggested patience as the new company got on its feet. In a letter to one director, Groseclose said: "Bryce has had so much to do since taking over this work that we all must be patient and helpful rather than critical of any mistakes that have occurred in the administration of our new corporation. The only criticism I have to make is that he is endeavoring to press the matter at so many points that he probably is not able to intensify his work at any one position in such a way as to guarantee success."[18]

At the October 11, 1939, board meeting, the board approved Twitty's request for additional office space, and the company subsequently took up quarters in Suite 209 of the same building. The board also elected Kimball as consultant with no salary.

There was a growing concern about "proper office systems." At the November board meeting, Wilson reported that he had spoken with Rufus Rorem, Frank Van Dyk and another executive of the Rochester (New

York) Plan, and they had recommended hiring someone to keep a closer eye on administrative detail. The board discussed the matter, and Twitty pushed for using the existing staff, as well as getting help from the staff of the International Business Machine (IBM) company to set up a system. Cary was named head of a committee of directors to investigate what should be done and report back.

Cary's committee on office administration made its report at the February 1940 board meeting, expressing optimism about enrollment growth and potential profits. At the same meeting, Twitty presented his administrator's report. Enrollment had grown from sixteen on August 1, 1939, to 35,125 members on February 20, 1940, (comprised of 20,662 subscribers and 14,463 dependents) from a total of 1,450 companies.[19] The company had received 171 signed contracts from hospitals, which accounted for 75 percent of beds available in the general hospitals of Texas. The company was now serving all areas of the state except in the Fort Worth and El Paso areas. (The geographic distance of El Paso made enrolling subscribers a problem, with a high acquisition cost. Fort Worth, though certainly close geographically, already had individual plans in two of their major hospitals. Twitty recommended that service be extended to these areas once the overall company was strengthened, probably in about two years.)

The optimism of both reports, however, soon yielded to the rising concern of the company's finances. The company had been in a deficit position since the beginning, and things were not getting better. Poor accounting procedures seemed to be part of the problem. In April the executive committee invited proposals from several accounting firms for audits on a quarterly basis. Nelson and Nelson of Dallas was chosen. By August 1 the accountants had not yet released their report, but they gave Groseclose enough information to sound an alarm, which he promptly did in a letter to each board member. Expenses, he said, were entirely too high and beyond initial expectations. He suggested closing several area offices, making "every employee of the corporation a producer—area managers will become salesmen."

At the executive committee meeting on August 5, J. R. Nelson of the accounting firm was present. Groseclose reported on his and Cary's decision to employ an auditor. Nelson suggested that while some expenses of the company were in line for such a new company trying to get a foothold, others were not. He said the company should reduce administrative expense by at least thirty-five hundred dollars a month. The board also instructed Twitty to seek less expensive office rental, even if it meant leaving downtown.

The next week Twitty submitted a report that showed reductions amounting to an estimated $1,694 per month. This included various office efficiencies, moving to cheaper quarters, consolidating the Longview and Tyler offices, employing stricter enrollment procedures, reducing some of the salary perks to salesmen that Twitty had originally promised, reducing the car allowance, and in some places cutting personnel, including a "special representative" at Lufkin who was causing a significant drain to the tune of three hundred dollars per month. (He was the brother of board member Jolly. In the same meeting a resolution was drafted and passed that prohibited employing relatives of board members or other employees. This was to solve the growing problem of board members recommending friends and family.)

Groseclose insisted that a claim department be set up. Twitty responded by saying that he would open a claim department with the venerable Kimball in charge of it.

Finally, the meeting ended with Groseclose announcing that the finance committee would meet to prepare a budget limiting the expenses of the administrator. Clearly, the board was taking a more assertive role in managing the young company, with Cary and Groseclose in the lead. Twitty's star began to dim.

The full board met on August 28 at the Athletic Club in Dallas. The board gave Cary increased authority, mandating that he, in consultation with the administrator, could reduce staff or expenses as needed, with the intent to put the company on a solvent foundation by October 1, 1940—just one month away.

On October 10, 1940, Twitty resigned as administrator, announcing that he was going to Hillcrest Memorial Hospital in Tulsa, Oklahoma. He and a group of investors were purchasing the bankrupt hospital. It is likely that earlier in the year Twitty had seen his role coming to a close and had been working on the deal for some time.

Groseclose immediately conferred with members of his executive committee and, after getting a majority opinion from them, asked Kimball to step in as administrator on a temporary basis at a salary of three hundred dollars monthly.

Although it is true that Twitty was a much better promoter than administrator, he went on to a successful career in Tulsa, staying in that job until his death in 1961. While his handle on details was loose, his enthusiasm for the potential of group hospitalization never wavered. His energetic vision for the concept that he had helped Kimball to launch eleven years before at Baylor remained with him to the end of his employment with GHS. He sent a letter to his hospital colleagues announcing the situation:

> A very fine, ultra-modern 225-bed hospital at Tulsa, Oklahoma has, for
> several months, held a very attractive offer open for me at a salary that I cannot
> turn down, and you know my heart is in the hospital work. Having Group
> Hospital Service, Inc., out where it will carry itself....I feel that the plan will
> grow with increased rapidity, and should have no trouble whatever in soon
> passing the fondest expectations of all of us who have been so vitally interested
> in it. Let's urge business men to join with the hospitals of Texas to make it
> possible for their employees to have this service.[20]

In mid-October just a few days following Twitty's resignation, the
company moved from the suite in the Medical Arts Building to a larger
space at 2022 Bryan Street. The white two-story building was on the
southwest corner of Bryan and Olive. It was a serviceable and unpreten-
tious office and afforded increased space at a reduced rental. It provided
a home for the young company for the next six years.

Kimball settled into his task as administrator. He recruited Annie
Laurie Surratt in early 1941 to be his secretary. She was the daughter of
Kimball's friend, John Surratt of the Kessler Plan Association. She had
substituted for two weeks as Kimball's secretary during his tenure at Baylor
Hospital.

At the next board meeting following Twitty's resignation, Kimball
presented his administrator's report. The last paragraph of his report described the need for the organization (especially the area offices) to shift
from a "promotional campaign organization" to one "of a more permanent type":

> (I)n this promotional campaign no more brilliant record in Texas insur-
> ance has ever been achieved than that that was made in the history of our own
> organization by Mr. Bryce Twitty and the various area managers. However,
> there are many economies of administration in handling certain parts of the
> territory that may be achieved by modifying this promotional organization to
> one of a more permanent type and by the readjustments of costs and personnel
> and budgets thereunder. At present, with our present set-up, there are many
> instances of duplication of work and other conditions that are not adequately
> reflected in economy or efficiency of results.[21]

Financial realities

Finances remained at the forefront of Kimball and the directors' concerns. The year-end financial results of GHS were sent to the Board of
Insurance Commissioners in Austin, showing a deficit of $48,881. The
board obtained a loan from a Dallas bank of $50,000, but the insurance
commissioners would not accept a loan as evidence of having relieved
the deficit.

The directors discussed the need for an experienced executive director of the company. However, it was difficult to attract qualified candidates because of the six thousand dollar annual cap on salary mandated by law. Most associate directors in other Plans across the country, which would be the logical place to fish for an administrator, were already approaching that salary. The Texas Plan could hire a younger, inexperienced administrator, but it was felt that the company now needed the experience. Rufus Rorem advised in a letter:

> The task of administering the statewide Plan in Texas is one as great as any in the country, and will need all the resources of experience and maturity which you are able to find in a single individual. It is no easy job to administer even one plan in a community with three or four hundred thousand inhabitants. It will be still more difficult to coordinate the regular activities in four communities of this approximate population, with a dozen other cities of one hundred thousand throughout the state.[22]

The committee on office administration and finance decided to call in Ray McCarthy, head of the St. Louis group hospitalization plan, to consult and advise GHS. That plan had agreed to lend McCarthy out at no expense except for travel allowances.

McCarthy came to Dallas, met with Groseclose and the auditor, and returned to St. Louis with a briefcase full of facts. He submitted a report, and Groseclose gave Cary an advance copy of it. "I am convinced that two things are wrong with our corporation," Groseclose said. "First, our plans; and second, our personnel. By this I do not mean that anybody is crooked, but I do believe that we are incompetent with our present set-up to handle this vast volume of business. It is the opinion of Mr. Nelson and Mr. McCarthy that a radical reorganization must be effected immediately."[23]

The executive committee met on June 13 and heard McCarthy's report. McCarthy suggested that the Texas Plan conform to standards set up by the AHA for Blue Cross Plans. He recommended that the company hire an experienced administrator and suggested Edward Groner, managing director of the New Orleans Hospital Service Association. McCarthy cited the weaknesses of the company: "The very fact that this great social movement was born in Texas, and particularly in the city of Dallas, really acted as a hindrance to eventual success. Your leaders in the hospital field and in the medical field contributed to the success of plans elsewhere by providing statistics and advice whenever called upon. Unfortunately, someone failed to realize that the Texas plan would be advantageously served by accepting advice from other citywide and statewide programs that were rich in experience. You were not privileged to take advantage of mistakes made elsewhere."[24]

He suggested a wide-ranging list of remedies:

- Reduce the number of area offices to major metropolitan centers;
- Put sales personnel on salary, not commission;
- Separate sales and service personnel;
- Enroll groups only;
- Pay hospitals on a service basis instead of merely reimbursing expenses, making the hospital guarantee the services of GHS.

The full board met the next day and heard the report. Kimball responded that he did not agree with all phases of the report, but the good of the corporation was his goal and he would do whatever the board wished. If the company abided by the report, however, it would require the services of a "young, active" administrator, and he did not feel up to the job. The board later offered laudable remarks about Kimball's service.

Groner was then invited to come to Dallas. He said he would like to come to Texas and study the Plan before agreeing to the job. He thought perhaps he could obtain a one-year leave of absence from New Orleans for the task. Groner made a preliminary visit, conducting a detailed survey of home office records and procedures, and visiting the area offices around the state.

On June 28 Groseclose and Groner attended the THA board of trustees meeting in Waco. Groseclose reported that the company was not faring well and told of McCarthy's visit and Groner's detailed survey of operations and the possibility of Groner coming to Texas. He asked the THA board to endorse three points in principle:

1. Liquidate the GHS deficit by having hospitals absorb whatever amount necessary to satisfy the insurance department.

2. Put hospital payments on a per-diem rate.

3. Completely reorganize the Plan, including canceling perhaps forty thousand contracts that were enrolled without sound procedures.

The THA board agreed to the points unanimously. The meeting was a most significant event in the history of GHS. If THA had not supported GHS, chaos could have erupted, probably causing the statewide Plan to dissolve. Now, with the strong backing of Texas hospitals, the company had another chance.

At the GHS board meeting on July 18, Groner delivered his report. The report suggested the three steps as discussed with THA, as well as tightening up subscriber contracts and internal office procedures and reducing the number of area offices. He explained that the most important step to save the company would be to get agreement from the hospitals to absorb the current loss, estimated by him to be as high as $125,000. Also, he suggested a general education program for the public, emphasizing the company's non-profit, service nature. He asserted that terms such as "policies," "premiums" and "insurance" made the company look like a commercial venture and that terms such as "fees," "dues" and "hospital service" should be used instead.

At the end of the report, he announced that the New Orleans board would not grant him a leave of absence to allow him to come to Texas. The board accepted the report, moved that 15 percent of all business done with GHS by the hospitals from the beginning, paid or unpaid, be absorbed by the hospitals, and approved the per-diem payment.

In light of Groner not being able to come to Texas, the office administration committee presented another candidate who had been invited to the meeting. The candidate was administrator of Group Hospital Service in Tulsa, Oklahoma, and had earlier helped McCarthy at the St. Louis Plan.

The candidate was Walter R. McBee. McBee said he would be willing to accept the appointment and could report to duty about August 15. He asked that his appointment be kept private for a while until he worked out things in Tulsa. It was moved and unanimously carried that McBee be appointed administrator of GHS.

Though the directors hardly knew it then, they had just inaugurated a twenty-six-year reign of growth and prosperity for the struggling company under the leadership of an extraordinary man from Tulsa.

4 | 1941-1943: Resetting the Foundation

*"I have never been involved in any business
failure and I don't cotton to the idea. I didn't
take this job to preside over a funeral."*
Walter R. McBee

On a sweltering July day in 1941, a confident man in
a smart suit highlighted with a well-chosen tie strolled into the offices of
Group Hospital Service in the white building at the corner of Bryan and
Olive Streets in downtown Dallas.

Euline Mitchell, the company's new receptionist, glanced up. "May
I help you in any way?" she asked, thinking he might be a potential new
member. "Hello, Miss Sullivan," the man responded mistakenly, having
been briefed that the receptionist was so named and not knowing that he
was addressing Sullivan's replacement. He then identified himself as
the new administrator of the company. Neither Mitchell nor any of the
other twenty-seven employees yet knew of the new administrator, Walter
R. McBee.

Although he wasn't scheduled to begin work until August 15, McBee
was in town to attend the GHS board meeting and a meeting of the Member Hospitals. At the meeting of Member Hospitals on July 19, the hospital supported the THA board and agreed to absorb GHS's losses.

McBee presented a striking appearance, always fastidiously dressed
and carefully groomed with wavy, prematurely grey hair that made him
stand out in a crowd. He was full of life and energy, often offering an
infectious laugh to any gathering. The flourish of his signature with the

pronounced curves of the "W," "R" and "B," matched the flourish of his personal style, but he was not flamboyant. He was always within the bounds of good taste, with a gracious style. Likewise, his wife Lillian was known as a woman who was quiet but not shy and always delightful company.

He came to Texas well experienced in administration of hospitalization plans. His most recent position was that of executive director of the Blue Cross Plan in Tulsa, which he helped organize. Before that, he was assistant director of the St. Louis group hospitalization plan.

Walter Raymond McBee was born April 22, 1903, on a farm near Advance, Missouri, where he attended elementary and high school. He went to St. Louis and accepted a position with American Credit Indemnity Company in 1921. While there, he took up the study of law and was admitted to the Missouri Bar on July 22, 1929. In St. Louis he was active in civic and community groups. He was president of "The Supper Club," a Toastmasters-like organization; a member of the downtown Kiwanis Club; and a member of the Masons, serving as Worshipful Master of Cornerstone Lodge No. 323, a Masonic Temple.

In 1936 McBee noticed newspaper accounts of a new hospital service plan that Ray McCarthy was organizing in the city. It interested McBee so much that he resigned from American Credit and worked for McCarthy for several months for free. McBee's wife even helped out at the office typing membership agreements, also for free. He finally went on the payroll as associate director.

In March 1940 he was invited by a committee of physicians to start a plan in Oklahoma. He and St. Louis Enrollment Director Harley B. West relocated to Oklahoma. McBee set up the corporate office in Tulsa and West became assistant executive director in Oklahoma City.

Why McBee chose to leave a comfortable position as executive director of the Oklahoma Plan and come to what was literally the frontier of the group hospitalization movement is unknown. He hadn't planned to move from Tulsa. In fact, he was on the verge of buying a home there. Perhaps he came to Texas because he couldn't resist a good challenge, which he certainly had in the Lone Star State.

McBee soon discovered that salvaging an existing plan was more difficult than starting a plan from scratch as he had done in Tulsa. Kimball was still active in GHS with a strong following, and, although he was willing for another person to take over, he was reluctant to turn loose of the company that grew from the concept he birthed. The Plan was broke, and the state insurance department wanted evidence of its solvency. McBee was not certain of the full backing of the board. Employee morale was low and continued employment uncertain. Some employees weren't quite ready to accept a new boss, particularly one from out of state. Enrolled groups were unhappy, and cancellations were high. Hospitals were losing their early enthusiasm. Competition from commercial companies was vicious.

Criticism was coming from out of state as well. Back in Tulsa, Twitty was wincing about the publicity given to McBee as a hero saving a broken plan and appealed to Groseclose to stem the "adverse publicity." Several doctors connected with the Oklahoma Plan were provoked by McBee leaving and were critical of the Texas directors who lured McBee away.

Bright spots could be found, however, in this otherwise dark horizon. Most significant was that the Member Hospitals agreed to absorb GHS's losses. This was a solid vote of confidence in the company. In addition, both the boards of THA and GHS had agreed with the Groner and McCarthy reports, which followed the principles set forth by the AHA, and leaders were looking forward to the day when GHS might meet approval as a Blue Cross Plan.

As McBee took office and began to survey realities, he worked hard at building alliances. He developed rapport with the board and struck up a warm friendship with Phil Overton, the company's lawyer in Austin. He also maintained close relationships with hospital officials because he realized that the hospitals not only formed the company but had also given it another chance with the decision to absorb the losses.

Cary and Groseclose put the weight of their influence and reputation behind McBee. Armed with that support, McBee went to work.

As he related to Overton in late 1941, the situation didn't look good, but McBee's natural optimism and enthusiasm for the challenge at hand, as well as his flowery prose, were readily apparent. He was faced with explaining an expected year-end deficit of sixty to sixty-five thousand dollars to the state insurance department. "If the figures go in as indicated, they will still look at us with those question marks," he confided to Overton. "We will, of course, not yet be able to show the public anything from the insurance department that will inspire their confidence, and believe me, we are constantly under fire from competitors. But let us be courageous, try to smile through it all, with the hope that ere long we will be able to smile at the thought that we were once worried, harassed, brow beaten and down trodden."[1]

The insurance department pressed the company for a more complete explanation of its finances and began to think about closing the company for insolvency. In December 1941 the department assigned two examiners to evaluate the situation and report to the insurance commissioner. The younger of the examiners was Tom L. Beauchamp, Jr, who had just graduated from the University of Texas at Austin with a law degree. He was an apprentice examiner assigned to assist the chief examiner but ended up doing most of the job himself. Beauchamp recalled, "The chief examiner was tied up; he hadn't finished the job he was on, and I was still pretty much of a greenhorn. He told me what to do to start the job until he could come aboard. I'd meet with him almost every day for lunch to tell him how I was doing and get answers to my questions. This went on and on, and he never did get through with what he was doing and get on this job. I completed and signed the examination report, my first full examination on my own."[2] The young examiner's first report termed the company's situation "chaotic."

Despite Beauchamp's bleak report, McBee used his charm to convince the state department that the company was salvageable. "I have never been involved in any business failure and I don't cotton to the idea," Beauchamp recalled McBee saying. "I didn't take this job to preside over a funeral."[3]

Reorganization

McBee and the commission agreed on a plan of action with monthly monitoring of the financial statement. The company had a reprieve.

McBee wasted no time in putting a reorganization plan into effect. The board granted McBee the authority to make changes in home office personnel without their approval. McBee then began firing seventy commissioned salesmen around the state. He hoped to save the expense of their salaries and to tighten up enrollment procedures by removing the financial motivation for enrolling anyone regardless of health. McBee wanted each of the nine remaining area managers to understand that their job was to enroll groups and not to manage commission men or to employ people to do the work for them.

Next, McBee and his staff began the task of canceling about twenty thousand members, many of whom had been enrolled carelessly. Many were not employed in a group but were random individuals and family and friends gathered to form a group. Others most likely enrolled while in ill health.

The remaining eighty thousand members were transferred to a new benefit plan that offered service on a per-diem basis instead of billing for separate services. Though in some cases this actually increased the benefit to the subscriber, it gave GHS more control over costs and made administration of benefits more efficient. Two coverages were offered: Service One provided a five-dollar private room rate, and Service Two provided a three-dollar ward service benefit. Hospitals were asked to sign a new contract and agree to the changes.

McBee kept in contact with Rufus Rorem, apprising him of the details of the reorganization in hopes of getting approval as a Blue Cross Plan. He told Rorem:

> In the beginning we canceled about twenty thousand persons and then were confronted with the task and in the face of competition of transferring all our remaining groups to the new service. Each member was required to sign a transfer card ... and of course the proceedings usually involved the necessity of a conference and sometimes many conferences with the executives to obtain their consent for the transfer and the continuation with our service. We have lost surprisingly few groups, but since they were scattered all over the state, it has been a tremendous job, requiring every minute of the time of our salesmen and depriving us of the privilege of obtaining new groups and of increasing our income. Most finished by December, but because of holidays it was the end of January before the work was completed.
>
> You can probably appreciate the state of confusion that has resulted during the last two months in obtaining new contracts from the member hospitals, to which the majority responded, and with a large portion of our members on the old service and the remainder on the new. Try as we may, the confusion was unavoidable and ran from our office throughout our membership and the hospitals. Naturally we lost some good will and some allegiance, but in spite of everything the cooperation and willingness to go along with us have exceeded my expectations, particularly since competition in Texas is active and decidedly keen.[4]

Employees worked long days, sometimes until midnight. McBee worked alongside his staff, moving files, stamping envelopes, doing whatever was needed. His expectations of himself and his employees were high. At Christmas in 1941, Helen Thompson let the office force go at noon on Christmas Eve. McBee later came out of his office to discover the building deserted. He asked where everyone was. "Mrs. Thompson let everyone off," came the reply. Given his nose-to-the-grindstone attitude, McBee was most likely angered, but he didn't show it, either then or rarely during the next twenty-six years.

That half-day off was one of the few fringe benefits of employment at GHS. Sometimes employees were paid overtime and sometimes not, depending on that week's financial condition. One employee recalled the hard times: "We were so poor at the time that we even had to furnish our own office pencils," she said. At one time the staff collected playing cards and sold them for scrap paper (which was becoming a wartime commodity) to get money to buy an office pencil sharpener.

McBee himself was no stranger to corporate frugality. With the new job, he inherited an old car—called "Martha"—that somehow got him around the state until the company could afford a newer model.[5]

Besides the hard times, the Bryan Street location provided plenty of other challenges. The plumbing continuously overflowed and ran down the stairs. Rain came in the back of the building. "The only way to keep dry," Personnel Director and Purchasing Agent George Dorsa said wryly, "was to put your feet on your desk." More than once, the employees recalled, drunks would come in off the street and pass out in the reception area. Some thought that they mistook the building for a hospital because of the sign on the front: "Group Hospital Service."[6]

Drunks weren't the only unwelcome visitors. The building had no air conditioning, so during hot weather employees would leave the front door open, and stray dogs often wandered into the building. McBee's office was on the second floor, and the staff kept dogs from wandering up the stairs to his office.

Throughout these business challenges, McBee was a hard worker, energetic and personable. Annie Laurie Surratt became his secretary until 1945 when she became director of the Case Department. (Because of her proficiency with numbers, she prepared the statistical information for board meetings and became the company's first actuary. In 1950 she was given the title of "Statistician."[7])

The picture at the end of 1941 was not positive. The Plan was down to 80,330 subscribers and dependents with an income of $45,375. The year-end deficit was $35,889 and, when added to the $71,000 hospital deferments, created a true deficit of $106,884.

As 1942 dawned, McBee was ever hopeful that his efforts would show results. "With the closing of this month," McBee reported to Overton, "we will have just broken away from our shackles and have before us an open field for a clear run toward the goal of earning surpluses and an improvement in our financial condition as a result of our operating experiences.... Frankly, I can see a clear road ahead for the year and feel quite optimistic and enthusiastic, but just how many people will see with me I don't know."[8]

In addition to the focus on financial and operational recovery, the company worked to achieve approval as a Blue Cross Plan by the AHA. When McBee came to Texas, one of his objectives was to get this approval. One of the first things he did was to have the company letterhead redesigned, sporting the outline of a cross but without the AHA insignia in the center. In this way he tried to communicate that this was a plan designed as a Blue Cross Plan but not yet approved as such.

Hopes were also high at the national level that GHS could become Blue Cross in Texas. "A couple of days ago Ed Groner in New Orleans telephoned me," McBee told Overton. "He had just returned from New York, where he attended a conference of the commissioners.... He also added that all of the commissioners and (AHA) trustees who were in attendance expressed much interest in Texas, including the hope that we will have our plan in condition for approval by the first of the year. I think, at least I am hopeful, that we will not disappoint them."[9]

GHS applied to the Hospital Service Plan Commission of the AHA to get approval as a Blue Cross Plan in Texas. The commission met on February 12, 1942, and decided that Texas was not yet ready. Responding to that disappointing decision, McBee wrote Rorem: "So we will just keep our shoulder to the wheel and work all the more diligently in an effort to have our plan in such condition as to remove any doubt when the subject of our approval comes before the commission."[10]

Blue Cross' fiscal health and standing in the community improved. The company assisted with festivities surrounding National Hospital Day in Texas on May 12, 1942, the birthday of Florence Nightingale. Texas Governor Coke Stephenson signed the bill commemorating the day with various dignitaries in attendance, including McBee.

As finances improved the company addressed the debt from Dallas business leaders that had funded the start of GHS. In July Groseclose happily reported to Ben Critz, vice president and general manager of the Dallas Chamber of Commerce:

> I am glad to report to you that the entire amount with interest has now been paid. As you perhaps know, the organization passed through some very dark and troubled days. But under the able management of our board of directors and our present administrator, Mr. W.R. McBee, our corporation is rapidly coming to complete solvency. Any non-profit organization that can borrow $20,000 for organization purposes and return it in full in three years is evidently a solvent corporation.[11]

In October the AHA commission again met and considered GHS's application. McBee went to St. Louis to be available to the commission for information. On October 19, 1942, the news came: The approval committee of the board unanimously approved the application of GHS for identification as a Blue Cross hospital service plan.

In Texas, GHS letterhead and promotional materials began sporting the AHA insignia in the cross, with the line, "The Texas Blue Cross Plan."

McBee presented the year-end 1942 financial report at the February 17, 1943, board meeting, which showed (finally) a surplus of $71,308. The corner had been turned. Enrollment remained down because of the cancellation of bad business. Administrative expense was up because of the planned restructuring of the company, but hospital claims were down, helping to boost the surplus. With financial recovery in sight, McBee suggested that the company begin repaying its obligations. He recommended, and the board approved, that the company repay 20 percent of the hospital deferment.

Later in the year, Groseclose's health began to wane. On the evening of May 9, he was driving home to Oak Cliff from First Methodist Church in downtown Dallas, where he had been master of ceremonies for the graduating exercises of the School of Nursing of Methodist Hospital. In the car with him was his wife, along with a nurse and her mother. Driving under the triple underpass just outside downtown, he slumped over the wheel and the car lost control, finally coming to a rest after jumping a curb and hitting a street light. An ambulance rushed him to his own Methodist Hospital, where he was pronounced dead on arrival.

History would give McBee the credit for rescuing GHS, but it was the gentle but tenacious leadership of Groseclose that guided the company during its first four years through its very dark days as well as its recovery.

In the shadow of his death, a special board meeting was called to elect Cary board president. With Cary's connections to the state medical profession, McBee would be able to take the next step of his revitalization plan: forming a companion company to provide benefits for medical and surgical expenses, adding a Blue Shield to the Blue Cross.

5 | 1943-1945: Creating a Companion Company

> *"I am having trouble batting down a*
> *wild idea of a couple of people."*
> Walter R. McBee

At a special board meeting on June 2, 1943, the board unanimously elected Cary as the new board president. Cary was very well known in Dallas and across the nation. He had been president of the American Medical Association (AMA) from 1932 to 1933, and in Dallas he was instrumental in furthering medical education, serving as the volunteer dean for the Baylor School of Medicine for many years and later helping form Southwestern Medical School. Also a good business-man, he built the majestic Medical Arts Building in downtown Dallas, where GHS had leased its first office. As the decade of the 1940s pro-gressed, he became a prominent national foe of the Wagner-Murray-Dingell Bill that sought to establish a nationalized health insurance system.

Cary was influential in the early-to-mid 1940s as it became evident that Blue Cross would have to sell coverage for physician services to meet market demand. Organized medicine was ambivalent about such companies in Texas and elsewhere, and Cary helped convince them that a companion company to sell medical-surgical benefits was a good thing for physicians as well as patients.

That Blue Cross was a good thing for the people of Texas was becom-ing very clear. At the same board meeting in June, McBee suggested that the company pay back an additional 30 percent of the hospital deferments. The board agreed, and the next year the remainder of the deficits was cleared. Hospitals were certainly happy over the progress of the company, quipped one board member, since most of them didn't think they would ever be paid back.

At the same meeting, the board agreed to McBee's suggestion that six director seats be added. One of those went to Lawrence Payne, who had left Baylor Hospital in 1938 for Waco. Shortly after his nomination to the GHS board, he returned to Baylor as administrator. Another director slot went to Tol Terrell of Harris Memorial Methodist Hospital in Fort Worth. Terrell moved to San Angelo in 1948 as administrator of Shannon Memorial Hospital. Another well-known Fort Worth businessman, W. E. Justin, was added to the board. Though Justin's tenure on the board was short (he resigned on March 17, 1948), his nephew, John Justin, later enjoyed a prodigious board career.

In May 1943 the state increased the 15 percent administrative expense ratio to 20 percent. The salary cap was also removed, and the board approved a salary increase for McBee: from six to ten thousand dollars.

In April 1944 benefits for all members were enhanced in an attempt to increase enrollment. This liberalization of benefits provided for full coverage for employed female subscribers (they had been paying a per-day surcharge while in the hospital) and removed some restrictions on care for certain conditions (such as venereal diseases, pulmonary tuberculosis, alcoholism and drug addiction, care in mental hospitals and elective vasectomies).

In the Fifth War Loan Drive (June 1944), the company's finance committee purchased thirty-six thousand dollars of war bonds and used the moment to testify to the strength of the Blue Cross Plan with public fanfare. "Daily the Plan receives expressions of gratitude from employers and employees for the quality and expediency of the service that is being rendered," one company newsletter stated. "They have learned from experience that this protection is 'as good as it sounds.'"[1]

McBee wanted very much to be able to serve the rural communities of Texas. In July 1944, the company enrolled the Texas Farm Bureau, comprised of farmers across the state, and for many years the Farm Bureau was the company's largest group.

With the company on a firm foundation, Payne (by now the administrator of Baylor Hospital) lobbied for the closure of his hospital's historic hospitalization plan with the transfer of members to the Blue Cross Plan. He explained that out of a desire to support Blue Cross, Baylor University Hospital had discontinued its hospitalization plan and was urging members to enroll with Blue Cross. The Baylor Plan ceased operation on

December 31, 1944.

To get in step with the emerging national Blue Cross movement, McBee requested in 1945 that his title be changed to executive director, which the board approved.

Adding medical-surgical benefits

As early as 1941, word came from the field that there was a growing demand among customers for coverage of physician charges in addition to hospital coverage. "The way things look I am going to lose a large group (over 60) in the Valley because they want surgical," reported a San Antonio salesman to McBee.[2] "We may also lose Bordens and a few others here because the employers...want employees to have full coverage." He suggested working out a deal with a commercial carrier to provide medical-surgical coverage.

At first McBee was cool to the subject because he felt that offering physician benefits would require cooperation with hospitalization so that only one payroll deduction could be taken. "I hope you will now forget this whole subject," he said.[3] McBee wanted to add medical-surgical benefits at some point but not in the middle of his reorganization of GHS.

A fledgling medical plan sponsored by the Dallas County Medical Society was already in existence in the Dallas area. It began operation on July 1, 1940, and required that applicants have a limited income to join: $2,000 per year for a single person and $2,500 for a married person. Although it included employees of the Dallas Ford Plant and the Neuhoff Brothers Packing Company, it was a small plan, reaching a maximum enrollment of only about six hundred subscribers. Dallas doctors never fully supported it, and the income limits severely restricted enrollment.

By 1943 McBee pushed for the development of a company that would work closely with GHS, realizing its marketing necessity. Consumer demand and the threat of socialized medicine were the forces propelling the development of these plans in Texas as elsewhere.

Consumers were beginning to want coverage for physician services, having seen how prepaid health care worked for hospitalization. In part, the existence of Blue Cross created a market for medical-surgical coverage. The commercial companies, unable to compete with the guarantee of services by hospitals (versus traditional indemnity payment for hospital service), had countered with the addition of medical-surgical benefits, thus furthering the development of nonprofit Plans.

The threat of socialized medicine also spurred the growth of medical plans on the 'voluntary' approach. The Wagner-Murray-Dingell Bill was introduced in Congress in 1943 with the purpose of establishing a compulsory system of hospital and medical coverage for all Americans. Though the bill never passed, it was debated and discussed for the rest of the decade.

In other parts of the nation as well as in Texas, the hospitalization plan was precluded by law from offering medical and surgical services, so a separate company had to be organized. Within GHS the question of the day was how to organize this new company. Another San Antonio salesman approached McBee about a medical-surgical plan. This time, instead of suggesting using an existing commercial company to sell physician benefits, he suggested starting a profit stock company, with profits going to stockholders but giving GHS the benefit of increased enrollment.[4] McBee counseled against a for-profit approach:

> If and when it does become necessary to organize such a company on a stock or similar basis, it seems to me that a better appeal could be made to the people if there were no profits in the organization. The doctors would provide the original capital with the understanding that the capital would be repaid out of earnings and they could be paid a good rate of interest on their investment. I think they will have to come to the point of thinking of service to the people and in terms of service to themselves rather than for a profit in addition.[5]

The San Antonio salesman got the idea of a stock company from a GHS board member of that city, John H. Burleson, M.D. Burleson continued to push for the profit approach and convinced several other directors, including the venerable Cary and McBee's trusted ally, Phil Overton. Burleson's persistence frustrated McBee. "I am having trouble batting down a wild idea of a couple of people," he confided to board member Margaret Hales Rose.[6]

McBee had demonstrated his business acumen in husbanding GHS back to fiscal health. Now, he would have his second challenge—herding a divergent board with conflicting ideas in the same direction.

"I am terribly sorry that these fellows have this wild idea as a money-making proposition," he told one hospital administrator confidentially, "because everybody knows that Group Hospital Service has had enough difficulties without adopting another undernourished stepchild in swaddling clothes to further sap our strength. Anyway, I just will not be connected with anything, at least will not be a party to or condone the inauguration of a program on such a weak foundation and that would probably destroy the confidence of our hospitals and the people with whom we have worked so diligently in an effort to bring up the confidence that was once practically nil."[7]

McBee worked hard to convince board members of the non-profit approach. One way he did so was to hire an expert on the subject. On

February 1, 1944, Tom L. Beauchamp, Jr. reported to work. Beauchamp was the state insurance examiner who had completed the review of GHS in 1941. The state insurance department had promoted him to director of mutual assessment companies, which put him in charge of GHS's activities. Beauchamp had monitored the company financial statements and was well-acquainted with the intricacies of GHS.

McBee recognized that Beauchamp knew the intimate details of insurance law and could assist with setting up the medical-surgical company along the lines he wanted. "Tom Beauchamp tells me that he thinks the most practical procedure would be to organize under the mutual assessment laws," McBee told board member Tol Terrell. "Tom Beauchamp recommends that somebody buy one of these little mutual charters...then promptly convert it to a mutual assessment plan, and we would thus eliminate any thoughts of profit such as an idea that people might obtain from a stock company, even though it was operated without profit. Beauchamp ...knows all the angles down at the Insurance Department and is in a good position to steer us on to a charter that could be bought reasonably."[8]

He carefully finessed board members until he achieved a majority who agreed that the new company, to be named Group Medical and Surgical Service (GM&SS), should be a mutual non-profit company.

Besides the question of being profit or non-profit, many other decisions about the new company had to be made:

Should it be a surgical plan only or provide benefits for surgery *and* medical services? Some people expressed concern about not having actuarial information in the light of the well-understood fact that people would tend to seek medical care more often if they had prepaid for it. Some had suggested starting a surgical plan only and, once experience was gained, expand it to include medical benefits. Because of market demand, it was decided to press forward with both medical and surgical benefits.

Should benefits be provided on a fee schedule basis or on a guaranteed service basis (such as was true of Blue Cross for hospitals)? Because of the geographic magnitude of Texas and the herculean task of conferring with each physician and obtaining consent to enter into a contract guaranteeing comprehensive services, it was decided to pursue a fee schedule.

What should be the relationship between GHS and the new company? This was a vexing question in other areas of the country. In some areas the two plans maintained two separate boards and staffs but cooperated on some aspects of doing business. In other cases, the two plans maintained separate boards but had one staff. This arrangement worked when boards agreed but created antagonism when they did not. In Texas this was solved by formalizing the GM&SS board to consist of the GHS board but with the addition of six GM&SS-only directors (mostly physicians). So the GM&SS-only directors attended and participated in the Blue Cross board meetings, with the result that both organizations were well coordinated and harmonious.

The two companies were also administered together. GM&SS entered into an agency agreement with GHS, which allowed administrative efficiencies and one payroll deduction for enrolled groups.

Another question and challenge was the role of organized medicine. In Texas, as across the nation, the development of medical-surgical plans as companions to group hospitalization plans was problematic to physicians. Physicians and their professional associations were ambivalent. Some thought it advanced public health, some thought it a necessary evil to fend off socialized medicine and some wanted none of it, fearing that it was socialized medicine getting a foot in the door.

In 1943 the AMA encouraged the formation of medical-surgical plans if they were controlled by physicians. In 1946 the AMA established standards and an approval program extolling physician control, choice of doctor, preservation of the doctor-patient relationship and permissibility of premiums determined by income (which was not instituted by GM&SS). In similar fashion to how the AHA managed Blue Cross Plans, the AMA set up a subsidiary, Associated Medical Care Plans, Inc., to oversee the approval program and work with the new medical-surgical plans.

A growing majority of Texas physicians began to understand that these plans might be a bulwark against state-imposed socialized medicine. McBee counseled a Chicago physician, "Sooner or later, regardless of the administration that may be on the throne, we are going to have some drastic form of socialized medicine and health service unless we the people and especially the doctors and hospitals do something ourselves to remove the incentive by providing a means and letting the people do for themselves what the government proposed to do for them and at a much greater expense."[9]

Cary was instrumental in convincing Texas doctors of the need for the plan. In a meeting with physicians from the Texas State Medical Association in July 1944, Cary told his colleagues that their "affirmative approach" was needed to stem compulsory medicine. He said the only way such a movement could be stopped was by positive action on the part of the medical profession, the Blue Cross Plans and the various insurance companies in fostering plans for medical and surgical benefits.

Though the state medical association was assuaged, the group's leaders felt that they could not enter into a contract with another organization but did support GHS in developing the concept.

Fund raising for the new company

Since the state medical association did not want to organize a medi-cal-surgical plan, the hospitals once again stepped up to the plate. In January 1945 letters went out to Blue Cross Member Hospitals (from Earl Collier of Wichita Falls, chairman of THA's Council on Hospital Service Plans) with a plan for raising money for the new medical-surgical company. He asked hospitals to voluntarily give an amount based on ten dollars per bed. The amount was to be given with the understanding that the new corporation was not legally obligated to repay but that these amounts would be repaid when the new company could do so without impairing its financial soundness. By May more than sixty thousand dollars was raised. The top contributor was Cary's Medical Arts Hospital in Dallas, which gave five thousand dollars, much more than the sug-gested per-bed amount.

On June 5, 1945, GM&SS purchased a charter from the National Mutual Benefit Association (NMBA) for eleven thousand dollars, with the approval of the state insurance department. NMBA held a member-ship meeting. Its president, George H. Cottrill, presented 343 proxies and voted to approve the transfer of the charter, change the name of the corporation to Group Medical and Surgical Service, move the home of-fice to Dallas and increase the number of directors. McBee was em-ployed as executive director. (NMBA was first formed in 1905 and head-quartered in Sherman, Texas. In late 1934 the home office was moved to Houston.) With the change to GM&SS, NMBA members had agreed to have their policies taken over by National Life Benefit Company.

Since GM&SS had remained a mutual company, it was required by law to hold an annual meeting of all its members in which directors and officers would be elected. This was an unwieldy requirement for an orga-nization whose membership was to grow to hundreds of thousands. The requirement was circumvented by including a space on the application card for each subscriber to sign a proxy giving the GM&SS board the authority to represent each subscriber at the annual meeting. Remark-ably, the proxy was rarely questioned by applicants.

On June 19, 1945, GHS announced the formation of GM&SS by issu-ing a press release proclaiming "Double protection now available for Blue Cross members." GM&SS then enrolled its first groups: the em-ployees of GHS and Baylor Hospital. Other groups were slow to enroll in the new service, perhaps partly because GM&SS established stringent enrollment requirements in an effort to start the company on a stronger foundation than was the case in the early days of GHS. Payroll deduction was required, which was a problem for many companies of the era, with the result that the payroll deduction requirement was often waived. Few groups actually met the enrollment requirements of having 65 percent of a company's employees on the medical-surgical coverage. Benefits were adequate for the day, providing a schedule of medical and surgical benefits that included obstetrical care and an allowance of up to three dollars per day for hospital medical cases.

In 1945 the war was finally coming to an end, the Allied forces having been victorious. On May 8 President Harry Truman and Prime Minister Winston Churchill announced the end of hostilities in Europe, and the Allied Forces celebrated V-E Day. Following the atomic bombing of Hiroshima and Nagasaki, Japan surrendered on September 2.

During the war years, Blue Cross of Texas doubled its membership, which stood at 135,000 Texans as of August 1945, paid more than $1.5 million in hospital benefits, increased benefits to members, started a companion company to provide benefits for physician care and in general recaptured the public's trust after a shaky start.

As America was about to enter a new era of material prosperity and growth in the post-war years, so was GHS and its companion company, GM&SS.

6 | 1945-1949: Post-War Progress

*"I am confident that our days of excuses
are over and that in the future we will be able
to boast about our enrollments as other
Blue Cross Plans have in the past."*
Walter R. McBee

With the end of the war, Blue Cross of Texas began to enjoy the benefits of peacetime. Sales people found travel easier. The shortage of staffing eased off, with veterans returning and needing jobs. Some offices that were closed in 1941 were reopened.

GHS was stable financially and operationally. GM&SS was an actuality, starting on a very solid foundation.

Enrollment began to creep upward as more employers offered Blue Cross coverage, sometimes paying part of the cost and occasionally paying all of it. Even the famous Neiman Marcus of Dallas, "the world's most fashionable store," gave "the gift of Blue Cross" to its employees in 1946. Stanley Marcus, executive vice president of the Neiman Marcus Company, announced the addition of benefits at a store staff meeting. "Neiman Marcus believes that health protection makes for better employees," he said.[1]

Other large employers across the state followed the fashion of the designer department store.

The efforts toward enrollment, the continuing fiscal stability and McBee's well-honed sense of public relations all contributed to a growing sense of public trust in the company. Texas Governor Beauford Jester even proclaimed April 11, 1947, as Blue Cross Day. The proclamation noted how the national "non-profit, community-service idea of hospitalization" had originated in Texas in 1929. The proclamation raised the ire of some commercial companies. In their official statement to the governor, the president of the Dallas Association of Accident and Health Underwriters said, "We heartily commend you in setting aside a day in the year to emphasize the importance of hospitalization, health and accident insurance to the people of Texas, but we do think it should be done without discrimination against any licensed taxpaying insurance carrier lawfully operating within the State of Texas."[2]

By the end of 1945, GM&SS had enrolled 10,854 subscribers and dependents. In 1946 the board voted to return the first 50 percent of the money given by hospitals to start the company and later in the year agreed to refund the remaining 50 percent. This did much to enhance the reputation of both GHS and GM&SS. Everybody had received their money back in a relatively short time.

GM&SS was not yet known as the Blue Shield Plan. Around the nation some medical-surgical plans were beginning to use the symbol. In 1939 Carl Metzger in Buffalo, New York, was the first to use it. Metzger was searching for a symbol to market the Buffalo Plan and took the insignia of the Army Medical Corps, which used the familiar visual of the caduceus. In Greek mythology the serpent's ability to shed its skin represented the promise of healing and had long been used as a symbol of the health care arts. Metzger placed the serpent on a blue shield and thus was born the symbol for the new medical-surgical venture in Buffalo. Metzger generously encouraged other Plans to use the symbol.

In 1946 the AMA organized the Associated Medical Care Plans, Inc., a group that approved medical-surgical plans in the same manner as the Hospital Service Plan Commission did for Blue Cross Plans.

As a prerequisite to approval by the AMA and the Associated Medical Care Plans, GM&SS had sought approval by the Texas Medical Association (TMA). But TMA remained silent. The company pursued AMA approval, which was received in September 1946. On October 1, 1946, the Associated Medical Care Plans gave its approval. Finally, TMA passed a resolution at their annual meeting in May 1949, officially endorsing both the Blue Cross and Blue Shield Plans of Texas.

This reluctance to approve the company indicated the ambivalent attitudes of organized medicine toward the emerging Blue Shield movement in Texas as well as across the country. Because of their fear of socialized medicine, some physicians distrusted the movement, and yet, as the 1940s wore on, the medical community began to realize that Blue Shield might be the antidote for a nationalized medical system.

Harry Truman's surprise victory in 1948 pushed health care legislation to the front burner. The Wagner-Murray-Dingell Bill suddenly had a second life. The AMA fought back with a harsh public relations campaign against the bill. The AMA and other organized medical groups, though not completely trusting the new Blue Shield movement, nonetheless began to support it (and/or its commercial competitors selling medical-surgical coverage) as a much lesser evil than compulsory government medicine.

Cary himself was in the center of the AMA's counterattack on government medicine. His biography, *More Than Armies*, described him as a hero who led the country to save free medicine and the medical profession from a movement "to deprive American physicians of their rights to function as individuals in a free nation and to bring them all under the auspices and control of Federal bureaucracy."[3] Many other civic organizations opposed the bill, and eventually the public support weakened and the much-touted bill expired in both the Senate and House committees.[4] One thing that probably killed the bill more than any other was the overwhelming success of Blue Cross and Blue Shield Plans across the nation, not to mention their commercial competition. Clearly, the voluntary movement had won the day.

Membership challenges

Despite growing public confidence, Blue Cross of Texas was not showing the membership growth hoped for. "All of you know that in the past," McBee addressed the company's board in 1946,

> our Plan has not enjoyed the growth we desired. Of course, we were able to find plenty of excuses: There was the bad financial situation that we had to overcome and the resulting destruction of confidence among hospitals and the public, which required considerable time to re-build and re-establish. There was the unavailability of manpower and the inability to pay the price required for the manpower that was available. I write primarily to say that in spite of all the reasons of the past, either justified or unjustified, I am confident that our days of excuses are over and that in the future we will be able to boast about our enrollments as other Blue Cross Plans have in the past.[5]

One of his solutions to the enrollment situation was the addition of Colonel Harley B. West as director of enrollments. West knew McBee from the old St. Louis days, when both worked under Executive Director Ray McCarthy. West joined the St. Louis field force in 1938 while McBee was associate executive director. In 1940 a group of doctors visited the St. Louis Plan seeking advice on starting a hospital service plan in Oklahoma. McBee and West went to Oklahoma in March 1 of that year. McBee was at the corporate office in Tulsa while West assumed the position of associate executive director in Oklahoma City. Active in the National Guard, West was drafted into military service in September 1940 and served in the War Department General Staff in Washington, D. C. until he was assigned to overseas duty in the Southwest Pacific Theater, serving on the staff of General Walter Krueger, commanding general of the Sixth Army.

At war's end McBee summoned West to Texas. West had earned the rank of colonel during the war but would remain active in the National Guard, eventually achieving the rank of general. (He retired from Blue Cross and Blue Shield of Texas in 1969 as vice president of marketing.)

McBee's other strategy for boosting enrollment was the development of another benefit service: the Comprehensive Service. In February 1946 the board approved a revised method of reimbursing Member Hospitals, from per diem to payment based on hospitals' regular and established charges. This allowed for more flexibility in benefits so that the Comprehensive Service could be launched. The coverage was better, and the rates were higher: monthly premiums for an individual went up from seventy-five cents to ninety cents.

The major marketing project now became selling Comprehensive Service to new groups and transferring old groups to it, as well as selling medical-surgical coverage to new and existing groups. It was an administrative morass, West recalled.

> The complications were a nightmare for the employer, the field staff, as well as the internal departments. There was an "old service" literature and application card, with and without medical-surgical coverage; Comprehensive Blue Cross application card and literature plus medical-surgical literature and application in conjunction with Comprehensive Blue Cross; plus a transfer to the Comprehensive Blue Cross with or without medical-surgical; plus a payroll deduction card if required. In the next two or three years, a membership in the application card master file might consist of as many as five to six cards stapled together.... An efficiency expert would have had a stroke at the thousands upon thousands of hours consumed.[6]

Later, West noted, the company began introducing new coverage without transferring all the old to the new, a pattern still largely in effect.

With the addition of West and the needed expansion of the Dallas area field force, no room was left in the small building at Bryan and Olive. Office space had been a problem for some time. In 1944 the board had authorized McBee to seek larger quarters, but nothing came of it. In early 1946 McBee found a property at Snider Plaza in Dallas' University Park. It was a modern, two-story building soon to be completed with ten thousand square feet available for a ten-year lease—and it even included air conditioning. However, the board was concerned about the price and the long lease, so the deal was never finalized. Then, the finance committee of the board considered purchasing the Jones Building at the southwest corner of Live Oak and Hall for eighty thousand dollars, but negotiations broke down there as well.

A new home office

On September 16, 1946, the committee met at the Munger-Cadillac Building at 2208 Main to survey the property. The building had been built to house automobiles. It had been home to a number of service departments for car dealerships (including Munger Auto Company and Prather Cadillac Company) and served most recently as the city auto pound. The building was in the process of being remodeled with small offices at the front and large open spaces for a loft or warehouse-type operation at the rear. It really consisted of two buildings: one, five stories high, and the other, three stories high. The second floor was offered at $950 per month on a five-year lease. The finance committee agreed unanimously.

Beginning in October Blue Cross of Texas moved from the little blue and white building on Bryan Street at Olive to what seemed at the time as the big new building at 2208 Main. It was not a glamorous home office and certainly had its eccentricities. The weight of the automobiles had warped most of the floors so that some employees had to use their wheeled chairs to roll up or roll down to and from their desks. Several years later the company installed heavy IBM billing machines on one of the upper levels, but the floors couldn't handle the bulky weight of the machines, so they had to be reinstalled on the ground level.

In 1948 the building was finally air conditioned. Until then, employees endured the challenges of doing office work in the sweltering Dallas summers with fans blowing hot air and paperwork all over the office. "Fans were spaced around the room, blowing like a tornado. We kept a bunch of rocks around to weight papers down on our desks so they wouldn't blow all over the office," recalled Jack Buzbee who started in February 1948 as a unit clerk in accounting.

The building served the company adequately and economically for fourteen years. The building was taken over floor by floor as needed until the company finally occupied the entire structure.

The challenges of inflation

During the war the cost of health care had been held down artificially by wage and price controls. The cost of prepaid health care was also affected. Now, with the controls lifted, prices were going up—and so were consumer expectations about health care, which the Blue Cross Plans (as well as the commercial insurance industry) had helped create. Health care workers who were underpaid before the war now found themselves in great demand with higher salaries. A new infusion of capital in health care research contributed to a new spectrum of high-priced procedures and medications.[7]

In late 1946 the board noticed that hospital charges were increasing rapidly, and GHS's losses were mounting. As 1947 began the situation worsened. Though nowhere near the dangerous levels of the shaky finances several years earlier, the losses were of concern. The unlimited hospital services provided by the Comprehensive Service were climbing rapidly, particularly medicines. Administrative expense was also more than usual. The organization was growing rapidly, requiring more space, more equipment, more employees, more area offices and more field personnel. In addition, as a result of the transfer of groups to the Comprehensive Service and the addition of GM&SS, extra expense, lost production and administrative time were occurring. Clearly, some important financial problems would have to be solved in 1947.

The board began to study the high utilization and review financial and operating statements. The questions were raised: Should the hospitals help again? Could they accept reduced payment? Were the hospitals the ultimate guarantors of the Plans' solvency or not?

It began to be apparent that the company was growing beyond the tutelage of the hospitals. Everyone was reluctant to do the obvious—raise rates. McBee, fearful that the Plan would lose subscribers if rates were raised, convinced the board that a rate increase was not the answer:

> Even under present conditions we should be mindful that after all there is a maximum which the public will spend on a voluntary basis for prepaid health care, and when the price of care provided through voluntary means exceeds that maximum the public revolts and either becomes indifferent or welcomes a governmental program.
>
> I estimate that it would cost a minimum of $50,000 to increase our rates. Aside from the administrative cost of changing every record in our office, heavy demands would be made upon the valuable time of our field men, which might better and more advantageously be used in enrolling groups. Sight should not be lost of the fact that we are big business, that we are dealing with big business and that big business has come to look upon and respect us as big business. Then we realize that these big groups, industries and organizations as a result of a rate increase would have to do a tremendous amount of work in obtaining individual payroll authorization from their employees and many of their records would have to be changed and revised. We deal with these people;

we know that they would resent it. Therefore, I think we should seek another means to the solution of our problem.[8]

On the recommendation of McBee, the board approved some modest limitations on three categories of benefits that previously had been unlimited: operating room charges, laboratory services and drugs. These minor changes were not enough to solve the problem. Later in the year, with losses still mounting, staff consulted with employer groups and reported that almost all were in favor of a rate increase instead of a reduction in benefits.

Finally, at the executive committee meeting on December 11, 1947, McBee presented a proposal that increased rates in early 1948 from ninety cents to $1.10 for individuals on the Comprehensive Service, with similar rate increases across the board. The family rate was now up to $2.60 per month. The company's first rate increase would be effective March 1, 1948.

The board had finally bit the bullet. Never again would there be such a long, drawn out reluctance to face economic facts. This also marked a move away from the hospitals being the ultimate economic foundation of the Plan.

As the company's marketing and finances matured, so did the company as a modern workplace. At their December 1947 meeting, the board approved a retirement plan that would go into effect on January 15, 1948, to be administered by Southwestern Life Insurance Company of Dallas. Twenty-seven employees were eligible immediately. Later, employees were provided with group life insurance protection through Southwestern Life.

The Blue Cross Texas Federal Credit Union formed on January 27, 1949, and began official operation on February 14. Fourteen members joined, comprised of R. P. Bourland, Jean Bramlett, Lohmann Burris, Jack Buzbee, Mrs. J. H. Carson, Pierre Crosson, Kathryn Nokes Dean, Marie Hunter, W. Lamar Lovvorn, James. L. McArthur, Katherine Redd, William C. Sexton, George D. Spradley and Helen Thompson. Each of the charter members paid twenty-five cents as an "entrance fee."

By the end of 1948, the financial picture was improving. GHS had added $128,696 to reserves, for a total reserve amount of $250,028. GM&SS added $201,876 to reserves, now up to $315,852.

McBee introduced a proposal for yet another benefit service: the Preferred Service. This was approved in early 1949 featuring increased benefits and a more liberal surgical schedule with increased rates. He also recommended a limited service, priced lower and designed to reach groups in smaller and rural communities where a common employer did not exist. This was a first step in developing various plans to meet different needs. Most Blue Cross Plans at this point had a single set of benefits. Though a necessary and even groundbreaking step for marketing, it proved an administrative difficulty as it increased the complexities of operation as well as cost.

In September 1948 the company's first newspaper ad appeared in leading newspapers across the state as well as in the Southwest edition of the *Wall Street Journal*, a familiar media mix followed up to the present day. The ad touted the Plan's "pattern of democracy" in the voluntary nature of the Blue Cross movement and emphasized how the company solved the problem of health care costs on a sound basis that was "of the people, by the people and for the people." The ad also displayed a financial statement of assets and liabilities, assuring the public of the company's financial soundness.

As the company grew more sophisticated, staffing became more delineated. The company's first organization chart was prepared in June of 1947. West had been named assistant executive director as well as enrollment director. Four staff members comprised the next level of management: Pat Murphy, director of public relations; Tom Beauchamp, chief analyst; R.W. Dansby, office manager; and George Dorsa, comptroller. Later, Rex L. Tidwell became an additional assistant executive director, while also maintaining his position as regional director of the Houston area.

It was around this time that many staff members were hired who would move up through the company's ranks.

In 1948 R. P. Bourland was hired in the Service Department (which performed underwriting and marketing services). He retired from the company in 1974 as vice president of administration. Bourland hired a young college graduate, Eugene Aune, in 1949 as a clerk in the Service Department screening applications. Wallace Langston was hired in 1949 in the Hospital Services Department. He shortly became director of that department (later renamed the Case Department), replacing Annie Laurie Surratt who was made chief analyst and statistician. Langston retired in 1977 as senior vice president.

In December 1951 well-known Dallasite, Melvin Munn, was hired as director of administration and public relations. He was KRLD radio's top personality and also appeared on KRLD's new television station, which went on the air in December 1949. At Blue Cross he replaced Pat Murphy, who had been doing public relations work for five years and who had been McBee's secretary before that.

National organizing

As the grassroots Blue Cross Plans gained success and prominence, it became obvious that some degree of cooperation would have to be established on a national level. But how was it to be structured? The strength of the Plans locally made national cooperation difficult.

In April 1947 McBee reported on a movement to coordinate the activities of the Plans in order to achieve more concentrated efforts and results toward Blue Cross objectives. The United States and Canada divided into twelve districts. The Texas Plan fell into District IX in the southwest. N. D. Hellend, who was executive director of the Oklahoma Plan and had succeeded McBee in Oklahoma, was the father of the District IX organization. The district was to consist of work committees including the heads of major functional departments of each Plan, such as enrollment, public relations and administration, so that each work unit in each Plan could come together and solve mutual problems.

Another challenge propelling national cooperation was the handling of national accounts. The hospitalization of members of one Plan in the hospitals of another Plan in a different state was becoming a problem, aggravated by increased post-war mobility of Americans. Admission to an out-of-state hospital could be troublesome, since the hospital needed some verification of membership. Another problem was the level of benefits to be provided. Benefits varied widely between the Plans, as did hospital charges.

As unions became interested in health coverage as a fringe benefit, the issue became even sharper because in some cases it was difficult for a national union to negotiate with myriad Blue Cross Plans when they could more easily go to just one commercial company. A "reciprocity" plan existed that was makeshift and problematic as it required each Plan to provide its own benefits to the member of another Plan so that lower-cost Plans were penalized by higher hospital costs in other areas. Upon the admission of an out-of-state Blue Cross subscriber to a Texas hospital, the hospital sent a notice to the Texas Plan. The company then wired or air mailed a letter to the home Blue Cross Plan, and that Plan then notified the hospital of the benefits the patient was entitled to. It was hardly an efficient system.

The Inter-Plan Service Benefit Bank was the next attempt at better coordinating national accounts. Developed by the Blue Cross Commission in Chicago, it offered an improvement over the old reciprocity system since it provided a mechanism to equalize the per-case cost between the Plans. It also offered a process to wire eligibility and benefit information from one plan area to another. It was a pilot project in 1947 and was formally adopted in 1949.

The Inter-Plan Bank idea proved successful. As the decade of the 1940s came to a close, McBee reported that fifteen Plans had cooperated in the enrollment of Bethlehem Steel, U. S. Steel and Laughlin Steel and that about forty-five hundred of those employees were in Texas.

A proposal to develop a national Blue Cross and Blue Shield organization to be known as National Blue Cross and Blue Shield Health Service, Inc., was developed. The plan was to superimpose Paul R. Hawley, M.D., a prominent retired Army Medical Corps major general, and a small staff on top of the existing Blue Cross and Blue Shield organization. In Texas as elsewhere, there was much suspicion about becoming part of a national organization, and the board tabled the matter. McBee thought that the proposed national organization would make Blue Cross and Blue Shield Plans like a national commercial company. Ultimately, the fear of losing local control and the local relationships between hospitals doomed the proposal.

However, it would be inaccurate to say that McBee and the Texas Plan were parochial. The Plan took an interest and a leadership position in the association of Plans. In 1946 McBee was appointed a member of the Board of Governors of the national Blue Cross Commission.

As McBee rose in national prominence, he decided to determine the exact location of the birth of the Blue Cross concept. Though Baylor was widely cited as the beginning of what became Blue Cross, a few directors of other Plans disagreed and thought that the birth of the prepayment movement predated Baylor. In fact, Baylor Hospital was not the first attempt at prepaid health care, but it was the first effort that was so successful and widely imitated that it evolved into a system of hospitalization plans.

McBee realized the need to nail down Dallas as the genesis of the Blue Cross idea, and he was aware of the positive publicity it would create, not only in Dallas, but around the nation.

In late 1946 McBee began writing officials of the AHA and the Blue Cross Commission about the possibility of honoring Baylor Hospital as the birthplace of the Blue Cross movement. "It won't get past the other Plan directors on the (Blue Cross) Commission," warned Public Relations Director Pat Murphy in a note to McBee in January 1947. "They don't have an 'originator' in their area, but bet they won't let us either."

McBee was willing to wager with the jocular Murphy. "I'll make you a bet that Baylor receives this recognition and will permit you to name the odds," he said. Murphy responded that a "well-onioned hamburger" should go to the winner. McBee upped the ante to three hamburgers, and the two agreed on a deadline of June 1.

McBee pressed commission officials, rallying his friends to the cause.

At first the commission avoided taking action, but McBee persisted and when it finally came up for a vote at the June 19 commission meeting, there was little opposition. The commission voted that "Baylor University Hospital, Dallas, Texas, be honored with the presentation of a plaque in appropriate ceremonies at the St. Louis conference in September."

Though McBee was ultimately successful, we can assume that Murphy won the bet and got her prize of the triple hamburgers, since McBee missed his June 1 deadline.

Officials gathered at the Statler Hotel in St. Louis on the evening of September 23, 1947, during the annual AHA convention. John H. Hayes, retiring AHA president, presented a bronze plaque to Baylor Hospital administrator and Blue Cross of Texas board member Lawrence Payne.

After Payne accepted the plaque, the outgoing chairman of the Blue Cross Commission introduced Kimball as the "father of Blue Cross." The 75-year-old Kimball advanced to the microphone to reminisce about how he started the fledgling that grew up to become a national movement. Once the plaque was back in Dallas, it was placed in the Truett Building of Baylor Hospital.

With the genesis of the national Blue Cross System of Plans thus affirmed, the Texas Plan continued to push for enrollment growth. West finally made his goal of 500,000 members on October 21, 1949. The half-millionth member was John J. Morris of Neuhoff Brothers, a Dallas meat processing company. Year-end figures were 531,127 Blue Cross participants and 285,317 Blue Shield members.

In the decade to come, the company would find itself growing more, maturing more and facing even more challenges.

7 | The 1950s: The Maturing of the Company

> *"We have become more business like. Our enlarged operations have forced this upon us. We will of necessity become more so. Don't let anyone put the idea into your head that Blue Cross is not still Blue Cross. ...We know what we're trying to do and we shall continue to try to do it—the Blue Cross way."*
> *Harley B. West*

In 1950 the number of employees in the Dallas home office had grown to 150. That was enough to warrant the creation of an employee manual. Illustrated with hand-drawn stick-figure artwork by employees, this first guide offers a snapshot of employee life at midcentury.

Employees had five paid holidays annually. Unlike some other companies of the era, Blue Cross did not schedule work on Saturday, so employees enjoyed a two-day weekend. Vacations could be taken only from May 1 through October 31.

The dress code was businesslike and conservative. "You were not hired to be a fashion plate," the manual admonished. "The girls will wear hose. The men will wear ties."

As was true of many companies of the era, the maximum working period during a female employee's pregnancy was the first five months; then she was terminated.

The Employees' Benefit Association provided for the purchase of gifts (for weddings and births) and flowers (for illness and death). This eliminated the necessity of continuous collections in the office. Dues for the association were twenty-five cents a month. Income from office vending machines went to the association, and members voted on how to use the funds for such items as ping pong tables in the lunch lounge.

McBee took great interest in employees. Service pins were given at regular intervals, and McBee insisted on presenting the pins personally. Even on matters outside of business, McBee would sometimes counsel employees. "If you have personal financial difficulties," the manual advised, "borrow through your Credit Union or seek the advice of the executive director."

The employee manual also reflected the company's service-oriented culture. "Together we render a service to the community," the manual stated. Further, it said that with hospitals and doctors, the company worked "hand-in-hand, to make it possible for the American family to secure and pay for needed hospital-medical-surgical care."

Blue Cross had a distinct vocabulary. The manual advised employees to say "membership agreement" instead of "policy," "monthly dues" instead of "premium," "hospital service" instead of "insurance," "hospital case" instead of "claim," and "enroll" instead of "sell."

As staffing grew, the company organization became more complicated with the organization chart showing an evolving level of department directors who were managing a level of managers.

By 1952 the employee count had risen to more than 250. That year, employees enjoyed a new snack bar. Working hours also changed that year, and company employees were allowed to vote on the preferred hours. They had been working from 8:15 a.m. to 5:15 p.m. with a one-hour lunch break. The majority (199 employees) voted to work from 8 a.m. to 4:30 p.m. with a thirty-minute lunch break.

Employee communications advanced as well. Since the late 1940s, employees kept up with company news in a chatty, biweekly mimeographed newsletter called *The Informer*. In March 1953 the first issue of *FAX* premiered. It was glossy, digest-sized, with pictures of company life lavishly spread throughout the crisply written articles. Munn had hired Robert Kimbrell in January as editor. Kimbrell took the pictures, did illustrations and designed the magazine. Volunteer "reporters" around the company submitted the articles. The magazine's name was developed through an employee contest. The first issue's cover showed one of the judges, Brents Broyles (formerly of Houston sales, who transferred to the Dallas area as regional director of sales in 1950), and Lottie Morris of the Service Department, who had submitted the winning entry.

As the decade progressed, so did technology. In mid-1954 the company got an automatic telephone dialing system so employees could dial each other directly. Before this system, an employee had to go through the operator to reach someone.

The company purchased an automatic check-writing machine in 1956, a "type 403 accounting machine" that was housed in the Machine Accounting Department. The machine required only one operator to turn out twelve hundred checks per hour for Blue Shield benefits, replacing three or four typists who had prepared checks individually.

In 1957 the company was the first Plan in the System to use the automated IBM Cardatype equipment. With the Cardatype an operator took information from membership applications and produced a punch card from which billing and statistical cards were prepared as well as membership agreements and identification cards.

The home office building got a small facelift in early 1953 with a modern-styled entrance. It was fashioned with a glass front set at an angle and a jutting overhang holding the commanding words "Blue Cross Building."

In general, working conditions at the company were advancing. Despite these workplace improvements, union organizers were attempting to unionize employees. In November 1955, without warning, organizers from the Office Employees International Union arrived early one morning and passed out handbills to employees as they arrived, pointing out all the benefits of union affiliation. Organizers were soliciting the signatures of non-management employees on a card requesting that the National Labor Relations Board call an election at the company. If a majority of non-management employees signed, the law required an election at the company to determine if workers would be allowed to join a union.

The move surprised management for there were no known employee problems of any consequence. McBee was wounded by the talk of unionizing. The election was held, and the union did not get 50 percent of those eligible to sign cards—77 voted for the union and 151 voted against. Elro Brown, a member of the board and an Oil Workers Union official (the one board member representing organized labor), resigned from the board in protest.

Enrollment strides

In the enrollment arena, the big event of the early 1950s was the introduction of the Catastrophic Illness Endorsement (CIE). Polio was the dread disease of the early 1950s. During these pre-vaccine years (the Salk vaccine was introduced in 1954), the disease was at almost epidemic proportions, particularly in Texas and the Southwest. The insurance industry sold polio coverage at a good clip, backed by much advertising and sales effort—and the public was buying. The commercial industry often preyed on the scare climate of the era—policies were overpriced and not always accurately described. Some hospitals were experiencing difficulties with certain questionable insurance carriers.

In June 1951 the company released the CIE. This rider covered polio as well as nine other dread diseases (leukemia, scarlet fever, diphtheria, small pox, spinal meningitis, encephalitis, tetanus, tularemia and rabies). The rider provided first-dollar coverage for up to five thousand dollars for two years after inception of the illness. The rates per month were forty cents for an individual and eighty-five cents for a family, far below most commercial competition that usually charged one dollar per person per month for similar riders. It was offered to all Blue Cross members. The rider required members to have both Blue Cross and Blue Shield coverage, so Blue Shield enrollment accelerated. By the end of 1951, 178,144 participants were covered under the CIE.

By 1954 polio became less fearful and less expensive to treat. Another disease began to command the public's concern: cancer. The company added cancer to the list of illnesses covered under the CIE at no cost to the subscriber and effective October 1, 1954. The CIE was extended to five years to better accommodate the time needed for cancer treatment.

The addition of cancer to all existing CIE memberships at no extra cost was thought to be the first cancer coverage anywhere. It was not a financial success, however, and the addition of cancer later required a rate increase on the CIE.

McBee reported to the board later in 1954 that the expansion of the CIE endorsement at no extra cost had caused widespread enrollment activities. He estimated that since the effective date, 87,615 had enrolled in Blue Cross and 96,489 in Blue Shield and that 166,164 members had applied for the CIE coverage.

Another first in product development was individual coverage that was inaugurated May 1, 1952. Several months before, the company conducted a non-group enrollment campaign for Dallas County only. The first member in Texas to receive non-group coverage in that pilot program was Juanita Edwards of Dallas who was enrolled in August 1951. A Non-Group Department was created in May 1955 to work the individual market, and Ray C. Ralph was named non-group coordinator.

Other new services that were rolled out in Texas in the 1950s include the "hundred series" that appeared in 1957. It offered three tiers of products that provided more options for benefits. The 200 Service was an economical product, the 300 Service a middle-tier approach and the 400 Service a top-of-the-line coverage. The 300 Service was the most popular. A supplement to the hundred series, the Extended Benefit Endorsement, was introduced in 1957 and was the forerunner of the company's major medical coverage.

In late 1958 the company introduced the Varsity Service for enrollment of college and university students. Under various GI programs, college enrollment had burgeoned and many of these students were married. While the college market never became large, it did demonstrate the desire of the company to serve all segments of the population.

Advertising the Blues

To support the continued introduction of services, the company began to advertise more assertively. The testing phase of individual coverage in Dallas County in late 1951 was the company's first major integrated advertising campaign with ads in both city newspapers and announcements on major radio stations. The newspaper ads ran every day for eighteen days and included coupons to send for more information. The spot radio announcements were broadcast on stations WRR, KIXL, KLIF and KSKY and invited phone calls to the Blue Cross Building. Staff wrote the ads and did the creative work.

The 1954 campaign announced the addition of cancer coverage and employed newspapers, radio and even one-minute television spots. For this campaign the company hired its first advertising agency, the Couchman Advertising Agency. In the one-minute radio spots, Melvin Munn voiced the answers to a customer's questions about Blue Cross and Blue Shield of Texas coverage. The spots played on thirty-six stations in eighteen Texas cities. In the television spots, McBee, West, Beauchamp and Medical Director Dr. Roy Lester appeared, explaining the advantages of the Blue Cross and Blue Shield service.

The first national advertising program for Blue Cross Plans was produced in 1953 by the J. Walter Thompson Advertising Agency of New York and appeared in *Life, The Saturday Evening Post* and *Look.* The Blue Cross and Blue Shield System was slow to use advertising, however, since Plans were non-profit community organizations. Some thought advertising was just too much of a commercial activity. But attitudes changed as Plans realized they needed to compete with the commercial health insurance industry.

In the 1956 national campaign, one ad featured a Texas Plan customer. Richard H. LeTourneau, vice president of R. G. LeTourneau, Inc., in Longview, touted the advantages of his firm having Blue Cross and Blue Shield of Texas coverage.

Besides advertising, the Texas Plan began using more creative and sophisticated communications to boost public awareness as well as sales. Packages of windshield stickers were sent to all groups for subscribers to affix to their cars. The stickers read, "In case of accident, notify Blue Cross." The familiar Blue Cross mark faced outward, a visible and significant advertisement as many cars throughout Texas began sporting the familiar mark.

National marketing issues came up again early in the decade, demonstrating the need for more national uniformity of benefits, enrollment procedures and rates among the Plans. The United Steel Workers' Union was on a long strike in 1950, and health care benefits became a bargaining issue. The executive director of the Pittsburgh Plan went out on a limb and promised the union a standardized health benefit contract for steel employees in Pittsburgh as well as in several other states, including Texas. The Texas increment consisted of thousands of unionized workers. The other Plans bought off on it, and this project became known as the U.S. Steel Syndicate. Several other steel syndicates were put into place in a matter of days.

Blue Cross milestones

In 1954 the Blue Cross concept marked its twenty-fifth anniversary. An anniversary flag adorned the front of the Blue Cross Building. "Twenty-five years is a pretty respectable age and certainly an indication of stability and maturity," counseled West in a memo to field staff.[1]

In cooperation with the Blue Cross Commission, Munn interviewed Kimball, Twitty (who was now in Oklahoma), Payne (the first employee of the Baylor Plan, who was now in Florida) and Frank Van Dyk (now enrollment director for the New York City Plan). E. A. van Steenwyk was interviewed by Donald Fairbairn, public relations director of the Philadelphia Plan.

In 1955 the company achieved two "million" milestones. On July 13, 1955, claim number one million was received for Mrs. Emmuel J. Roberts of Waco, admitted to Providence Hospital for a thyroidectomy. An ad featured her with the company's very first case, Richard Sledge Harvey of Tyler, now twenty-one years old and a student at Southern Methodist University. His claim was received in September 1939 (when he was five years old) for a tonsillectomy at Mother Frances Hospital in Tyler.

On Nov. 30, 1955, the company achieved one million members after more than a year of pushing toward that goal.

At the March 1950 board meeting, Markham stepped down as vice president, a post he had held since the 1939 incorporation.

The most noticeable loss to the board (and the entire company) came December 11, 1953, with the death of Cary at age 81. He left a legacy of accomplishments not only at Blue Cross and Blue Shield of Texas where he had been board president for a decade but among the medical community of Dallas and even the nation. The death of the "Doctors' Dean" was front page news in Dallas. Texas Governor Allan Shivers said, "I have lost a warm friend." Dallas Mayor R.L. Thornton lamented, "We've lost one of Dallas' greatest citizens." Other civic, medical and government leaders lauded Cary's accomplishments and mourned his death. In 1959 the city school district memorialized him by building E. H. Cary Middle School on Killion Drive in northwest Dallas.

At the next board meeting in March 1954, F.J.L. Blasingame, M.D., was elected president of the board. In 1957 Blasingame was elected executive vice president of the AMA, a position that included being general manager of the AMA in Chicago. He resigned from the board and was replaced as president by L. H. Allen of Houston. Blue Cross and Blue Shield of Texas had good representation with both TMA and THA during this time, as board member Tol Terrell was elected president of the AHA and took office in September 1957.

In the enrollment area, Francis Bolton became Blue Cross' first woman enrollment representative in 1951 and remained the company's only female sales person for many years. Hired in July 1948 as a secretary in Austin, Bolton was later instrumental in helping to penetrate the state employees' market.

In May 1950 a Medical Department was formed with S. P. Bliss, M.D., hired as the company's first medical director. Bliss resigned in early 1954 to take a position with the M. W. Kellogg Company of New Jersey and New York. Roy T. Lester, M.D., became medical director on July 1, 1954.

Justin Ford Kimball died in his sleep on October 7, 1956, at age 84. After McBee arrived, Kimball had left GHS and was elected to the State Board of Education in 1949 but resigned February 1, 1952, before his term was to end late that year. He wanted to revise his civics book, *Our City Dallas,* which was out of date. "I am now in my eightieth year," he said in his resignation letter, "and have in me probably one more place of creative work for the public; I know of no more worthwhile legacy I can leave to my city and its children than to rework and rewrite this book on a new up-to-date basis."[2] It was to this task that he wanted to devote his year. His revised book was published a few years later and enlightened a new generation of Dallas schoolchildren.

His death was front-page news in both Dallas newspapers, which named him the "grand old man of education" and the "father of Blue Cross." One Waco newspaper (Kimball had practiced law in Waco in the early part of the century) described him as "a great American builder" on the editorial page. "Justin Ford Kimball typified all that is good, all that is lively, all that is inspirational in our way of life. He blessed his native state in a way that few men ever do."[3]

To commemorate his legacy as a pioneer of Dallas educators, the school district built Justin Ford Kimball High School on South Westmoreland in Oak Cliff.

The Blue Cross and Blue Shield System, which had grown from Kimball's initial concept, paused as well to honor him. The Blue Cross Commission met in Dallas for the first time in December 1956 in recognition of Dallas as the birthplace of Blue Cross and in memory of Kimball. Dallas Mayor R.L. Thornton made a surprise visit during the opening session at the Baker Hotel, welcoming the delegation. During the meeting a wreath was placed on the commemorative plaque at Baylor Hospital.

In 1958 the Commission instituted the Justin Ford Kimball award to be given annually to a person who has "faithfully demonstrated his dedication to the aim first stated by the founder of Blue Cross." E. A. van Steenwyk, who fashioned the first use of a blue cross for the hospitalization plan in Minnesota, received the first Justin Ford Kimball award.

Mounting financial pressures

The cost pressures first felt in the late 1940s during the post-war boom continued through the 1950s. Financial pressures were mounting because of increased utilization of benefits, the continued rising cost of health care and even a small amount of price padding by a few hospitals and doctors. Part of the utilization difficulty was the addition of cancer to CIE in 1954. Expenses for the disease ran higher than expected. Cancer was very difficult to forecast since no reliable statistics about the incidence of the disease existed. Indeed, Blue Cross and Blue Shield of Texas became the prime source of cancer statistics.

Rate increases were one response to the financial pressure. Though still reluctant to change rates too often, the board voted a rate increase for Blue Cross in 1951. (Blue Shield rates held steady.) "Inflation finally got us!" exclaimed the *Blue Cross and Blue Shield Bulletin,* a monthly flyer sent to enrolled groups. "Just like the grocery bill, hospital services have gone up, up, up in cost. It just takes a lot more money to pay hospital bills than it used to!" Two months later, another *Bulletin* reported, "Thank you for the spirit and complete understanding with which you accepted your rate increase; the first since March 1948."

The company responded to these financial pressures with several processes that soon became commonplace.

Member Hospital contracts were revised to give the company more control over charges so that either the company or the hospital could cancel the contract with written notice. The process for approving Member Hospitals was formalized and expanded. Hospitals were required to furnish an itemized list of drug charges. Blue Cross representatives began making more frequent visits to hospitals to check charts and charges and to discuss mutual problems. Member Hospital audits became a standard activity. All this was the beginning of an extensive Hospital and Professional Relations Department.

This new stance caused concern among some hospital administrators and field employees. West admonished his field staff in April 1950:

> Recently comments have filtered in from hospital administrators and from old time field men to the effect that Blue Cross is not like it was in the old days. Cases are no longer approved without question, applications are not accepted without haggling, exceptions aren't made, hospital charges are questioned, additional information is asked of the doctors, waivers are asked from applicants with existing physical conditions. The tenor of these comments was that Blue Cross was not like Blue Cross used to be....

> We have become more business like. Our enlarged operations have forced this upon us. We will of necessity become more so. Don't let anyone put the idea into your head that Blue Cross is not still Blue Cross based on the rejection of a hospital case which should have been rejected, based on correction of a hospital bill with incorrect items charged to us, based on an application set up for the anniversary date which should have been deferred until the anniversary date under our regulations, based on requesting payment on a statement already past due. You, I, the Dallas office employees, and the board still constitute Blue Cross-Blue Shield. We know what we're trying to do and we shall continue to try to do it—the Blue Cross way.[4]

To drive home the point that the company was growing, interoffice memo forms in the early 1950s began to sport the phrase "Think Big! Act Big!"

One way the company began to act big was to improve communication with hospitals and doctors in hopes of holding down costs. McBee understood that both the Blue Cross company and the Blue Shield company in Texas had been originally financed by hospitals, and he felt a particular closeness to Texas hospitals that never wavered. In the early days, McBee himself had called on hospitals, but, with the expanding organization, this was no longer feasible. Rex Tidwell began working with hospitals in the southern section of the state. George Walters and Tom Starke were hired and traveled around the southern part of the state with Tidwell. In 1953 McBee hired Bob Hawthorne, administrator of Children's Medical Center in Dallas, to work with Dallas area hospitals. These men, and many others hired subsequently, would carry on the tradition of keeping dialogue open with hospitals to solve mutual problems.

Staff in the hospital and professional relations areas soon put together workshops and took them to hospitals across the state. The Blue Cross workshops were called the road show among staff. The workshops provided for discussions between hospital staff and Blue Cross staff on day-to-day problems. This activity was copied by other Plans with good results. With the Blue Cross workshops so successful, the program was replicated for a Blue Shield workshop with physicians.

The end of community rating

Perhaps the most significant result of working in a more sophisticated health care and economic environment was the abandonment of the community rating system. A new rating system begun July 1, 1956, placed groups in one of six brackets based on past claims history.

In the early days, community rating was a strong selling point since everyone paid the same. However, as time went by, it became obvious that the larger groups with good experience objected to sharing the poor experience of other groups and individual enrollees. Another factor leading to experience rating was that employers were increasingly paying the cost of employee coverage and so employers wanted to manage that cost with whatever tools were available.

Besides moving away from community rating, some groups were transferred to a lower benefit product. One such type was the community enrollments. Since the early days of the company, attempts had been made to enroll whole communities, typically smaller towns that could not support larger employer groups. As could be expected, some of these groups showed very high usage of benefits, and these groups were moved to the lower tier of the Standard Service. Gainesville was the first community enrollment, and records show enrollments in Mission and Perryton, and there were probably others.

The company also began an experiment in the Orange, Texas, locality. A twenty-five dollar deductible per admission was added to all groups that were running in the red. The first group to receive the deductible was a DuPont plant. West traveled to Orange to talk to the plant's supervisors about the deductible and why it was necessary. The group accepted the deductible. West recalls that this could have been the first deductible used in any Blue Plan. Discussion about deductibles had occurred among the Plans, but some Plans were reluctant because it seemed so much like commercial insurance. Eventually, many Plans began using deductibles. In 1953, with the experiment in Orange a success, the board approved introducing the twenty-five dollar deductible per admission in more areas and with more groups.

Another activity to better manage claim dollars came into being at this time. The company began coordinating benefits if a subscriber had duplicate group coverage that might provide benefits for health care. Before, if a subscriber had both commercial and Blue Cross hospital coverage, Blue Cross would tend to catch the full liability since it offered easy hospital admissions and provided service benefits rather than indemnity reimbursement.

The price of success

As Blue Cross and Blue Shield became more known and popular, company officials realized that success had its price.

Doctors constantly requested either increased or additional benefits. These requests did not sit very well with the board in view of the failure of the medical profession to give financial support or official recognition of the Blue Shield operation. A few medical specialties even sought recognition on the board, but the board took the position that members should be selected based on individual qualifications with no regard to specialty. This quashed the pursuit of special interests on the board.

Patients, too, were learning to take advantage of their coverage. A hospital administrator gave McBee a letter the hospital had received in 1953 from the husband of a patient:

> Because of the terms of my insurance policy, I can collect approximately $250 extra if I check Mrs.————out of the hospital and then right back in again next Sunday. If she feels up to it, I will call an ambulance, put her on a stretcher, take her out the exit, drive around the block and then bring her back in, provided that neither you nor the hospital has any objections to this procedure.[5]

The doctor responded that the scheme would be detrimental to the patient's health. It appears that the patient was covered by a commercial policy, but certainly this was indicative of a new level of public expectation regarding all types of health coverage.

Perhaps the most flagrant way others took advantage of the company was when some commercial companies marketed policies with names that sounded suspiciously like Blue Cross. The most noteworthy of these cases was the Blue Seal case.

A commercial insurance company headquartered in Dallas was marketing an indemnity health insurance product called Blue Seal in several markets, including Arkansas. Testimony showed that at least some sales agents played up the public confusion of Blue Shield and Blue Seal.

This became a national problem, and both the Blue Cross and the Blue Shield Commissions mobilized a large national effort. In June 1955 it was announced that a settlement and complete victory had been reached. The insurance company was instructed to quit using its Blue Seal name and logo as well as a White Seal product in another company owned by the commercial carrier. It was instructed that it would never use any mark involving the words or symbols of blue, shield or cross.

AHA obtained a federal copyright on the name Blue Cross and on the cross insignia. Copyright laws required that the ownership of such copyrights rests with an individual or corporation. The solution proposed by AHA was that each individual Plan assign its rights to the name and the symbol to the AHA, which in turn would extend the privilege of using them back to the individual Plans through a licensing agreement. Concern in Texas and elsewhere was that this was infringing on the autonomy of the local organization. However, it was decided that in essence there was little difference between the then-present use of the Blue Cross name and its symbol being controlled by the approval program of the Blue Cross Commission of the AHA. Plans quickly agreed to the change.

In 1952 McBee suggested changing the corporate name from Group Hospital Service, Inc., to a name including the term Blue Cross, such as Blue Cross of Texas, Inc. McBee's thinking was that no matter what happened nationally, the Texas Plan would have a Texas registered name and symbol. It was announced at the March board meeting that McBee had conferred with the Blue Cross Commission and that they expressed no objection to using Blue Cross in the legal name. However, this idea died because the fears disappeared that had been originally expressed. It rose again thirty years later when the corporate name was changed.

In 1955 the Blue Cross Commission proposed the establishment of five regional offices (with four in the U.S. and one in Canada). Though the District IX operating committee as well as the GHS board opposed the move, the commission proceeded, and one regional office ended up in Dallas. Despite the early opposition, any feared problems failed to materialize, and the cooperation between the company and the new regional office was close and smooth. In 1957 Joe Elliott, a member of the Dallas enrollment staff, was even selected to head up this new office that was housed in Dallas' new Mercantile Bank Building downtown.

The Blue Cross Association had been formed in 1949 as a national enrollment agency for member Plans. It began to take on some of the functions of the Blue Cross Commission, and soon the two groups had considerable overlapping and conflicting operational areas between them. A national committee worked on a consolidation of these organizations, which was accomplished in 1960 as the Blue Cross Association supplanted the former Blue Cross Commission of the AHA. Texas board member Tol Terrell was a member of this committee.

The Blue Cross Association was also the holding company for Health Service, Inc., of Illinois, a mutual insurance company chartered in Illinois in 1950 to help with national enrollments. George Walters left the position of regional director of the Midland office to join Health Service, Inc., in New York City, in May 1952. He had started in the Houston area office in 1946. He returned to Blue Cross and Blue Shield of Texas in June 1959.

As a precursor to national activities on a wider scale, the company served a promising piece of federal business in 1956. In June of that year the Dependent Medicare Care Act was signed into federal law, providing a health care program for members of the uniformed services and their dependents. (The more familiar Medicare for senior citizens came in 1965.) The Department of Defense allocated certain states to Blue Cross Plans and certain states to commercial insurers, trying to be fair to both sides of the health benefit business. Texas was assigned to a commercial carrier, but the defense department also asked state medical associations to select their own agent to handle the medical-surgical side of the business, and TMA selected Blue Shield of Texas. Within a year Blue Shield had paid one million dollars to Texas physicians through the program. In April 1958 TMA did not renew its contract with the government and so Blue Shield of Texas was no longer a fiscal agent.

Toward the end of the decade, the company was approaching five hundred employees. Employee growth mirrored a maturity gained in the 1950s and prepared the company for new challenges.

The company was about to enter a new era of growth. If, as West's admonition in the early part of the decade suggests, staff had thought of the company as a small entity, they would soon see themselves as associates of the Cadillac of the industry. The first move in that direction would be to leave behind the ugly duckling of a building on Main Street and to construct a gleaming skyscraper across the street.

The company would soon be big business.

8 | 1960:
A Living Symbol

> *"This new Blue Cross-Blue Shield home office*
> *building is a living symbol of the objectives that*
> *inspired years of planning and building."*
> *New building brochure*

The company was twenty-one years old in 1960, and in many ways the year marked the time that the company reached adulthood. Business was about to become big for Blue Cross and Blue Shield of Texas.

The most important event of the year was the long-awaited completion of new headquarters. Since the mid-1950s, the company had been outgrowing the building at 2208 Main Street. "This building was not even planned for office use," Beauchamp wrote McBee in 1957. "Even as remodeled for our purpose it lacks a great deal of affording the arrangement and facilities needed to accommodate our operations in an efficient way. Automation is the current keynote of progress in streamlined, low-cost processing of high-volume office work."[1]

In December 1954 a building committee of several board members was formed to guide planning for acquiring adequate home office space. The committee discussed the merits of either renting or purchasing a facility. At first, McBee was enthusiastic about some property on the campus of the Southwestern Medical Foundation, which was across from St. Paul Hospital and at the corner of Harry Hines Boulevard and Inwood. The committee seemed more interested in finding a location in or near downtown. A real estate agent was brought into the picture—D.C. "Dub"

Miller, who also served on the Dallas City Council with Beauchamp.

Throughout 1956, various locations around the city were considered. One real estate firm suggested building an eight-story building at North Central Expressway and Fondren Drive in University Park and leasing to the company. Another offer was for a twenty-story building with a façade of blue porcelain enamel accented by gold aluminum trim to be built in the 1500 block of Elm Street downtown.

Other property was for sale downtown, and the most attractive turned out to be just across the street from the current building. Several pieces of property were available across Main Street extending along Central Expressway from Main to Elm streets. The primary tract was from the Hart estate of the Hart Furniture Stores of Dallas. The largest portion of this property contained a public parking lot across the street. Some of the other properties adjoining the main tract included a tool and jewelry store, a grocery store and a barbeque café.

The location was desirable. It was considered near downtown, six or seven blocks to the east of the heart of the city. That brought the land prices down somewhat but still retained the central location thought necessary for the convenience of employees. Parking space was potentially available, and the property was inside the proposed loop of an expressway (the Julius Schepps Freeway). Beauchamp and McBee consulted with Dallas Mayor Thornton, who highly recommended the property and the location.

In 1957 the company selected the architectural firm of Thomas, Jameson and Merrill. They had designed several significant Dallas buildings, including the Dr Pepper Company's general offices, Truett Memorial Hospital at Baylor, a recent addition to the Titche-Goettinger store, Park Cities Baptist Church and the Church of the Incarnation on McKinney Avenue.

At first, the building committee envisioned a ten-story building but then decided it would not cost much more proportionately for two additional stories, which would also provide space to rent out. In July 1957 the board decided to proceed with a twelve-story building.

The company had purchased the land, hired the architect and prepared plans when the state insurance department questioned whether under existing laws it was legal for the company to own real estate. A company operating under the enabling act (Blue Cross and Blue Shield of Texas was the only company then operating under the act) could not include a building as an asset. The estimated cost of the building was to be more than $5 million, so this was something to consider.

It occurred to management that perhaps GM&SS could own the building, since it was not operating under the same code. However, Beauchamp determined that because GM&SS was a mutual assessment company, it was not lawful to construct and own a home office building either. Most Texas mutual assessment companies were small (although GM&SS was large and financially strong) and were designed to serve local situations. The legislature did not want the assets of these companies diverted into real estate rather than helping their policyholders.

Management found an answer—a rather unusual one. Another company would be allowed to finance the construction of the building and lease it back to GHS with an option to purchase at the end of several periods. The expectation was that in the future GHS would be financially able to obtain ownership without the need to show the building as an asset on the balance sheet. The first step was to invite mortgage and finance firms to bid on the financing at the same time as they bid on the construction.

Henry C. Beck Company was chosen as the construction company and as the owner of the building, which was financed by Glenn Justice Mortgage Company. Beck took ownership on July 1, 1958. The construction proceeded as if GHS was paying for it, and the architect remained responsible to GHS. (GHS finally purchased the building on July 1, 1970, when it was strong enough to carry the financial load without showing it as an asset.)

In April 1958 destruction of the existing buildings on the property began, and by July the property was cleared and construction began. By October the basement had been excavated, and the steel skeleton began to take shape.

Because employees were across the street from the new building, they were able to view the construction. On November 5 as E. W. Hahn, then manager of subscriber accounts, was waiting for the elevator, he turned to look out the window and spy on the progress of the steel skyscraper. He described what he saw at that moment: "I was just standing there waiting on the elevator when I saw, across the street, everything falling down. Something had happened."[2]

On another floor, Judy Johnson, secretary to the medical director, was also waiting for the elevator and looked out the window. "Suddenly there was a horrible crash and I saw that something had happened and it looked to me that it was at the center of the building. I first thought it was Lester Loftice. He was manager of building and Mr. McBee had him over at the new building most of the time with a hard hat so he would know everything there was to know about the building, like electricity and water mains."[3]

Loftice was not involved in the accident, but a worker was killed and two other workers were injured. The accident occurred when a load of beams was hoisted to the fourth floor level (as high as the structure was at that point) and slammed against a steel column. Though the column was bolted in place, the impact toppled it against another column, upsetting a stack of steel beams lying on a platform. Garvin O. Williams of Crandall was knocked off balance and fell to his death into the basement sixty feet below.

McBee was devastated about the news. Someone told him that according to statistics, one person was killed for every ten stories. "That doesn't matter to me, that wasn't supposed to happen with our building!" he snapped.[4] He had a meeting with employees to explain what had occurred.

Despite the tragedy, work progressed, and the building was nearing completion by the end of 1959. McBee had announced that the move-in would begin in December, but various delays on interior problems delayed the move until April 1960.

As the building took shape, the pride among employees rose even taller than the building's twelve stories. Just twenty-one years before, the fledgling company was struggling with only a few employees in a leased two-room office. It had grown to be the state's most prestigious health benefits company with a brand-new building.

Modern As Tomorrow was the lead headline in a brochure commemorating the new building. "This new Blue Cross-Blue Shield home office building is a living symbol of the objectives that inspired years of planning and building. It provides a final touch of streamlined efficiency and economy which only a modern building designed specifically for Blue Cross and Blue Shield could give."

The building was more than a building. It was, as the brochure copy indicated, a symbol. It was a monument to the idealism of the company, its employees and especially its executive director who was approaching the end of his second decade as the Plan's leader.

The twelve-story office building was located at the corner of Main Street at North Central Expressway. North Central at that location wasn't really an expressway—it was formerly Preston Street in downtown and fed into the freeway. A seven-story parking garage was attached on the north side of the building at the corner of Elm Street and North Central. The total land and construction costs were about $5.5 million.

The modern design was laden with exterior elements to showcase its streamlined nature. Red granite columns running from the bottom to the top emphasized the inner steel framework. Between the granite were columns covered with aluminum, which hid air ducts for the heating and air conditioning system. (Putting the ducts outside saved interior space.) Contrasting with these vertical lines were deep horizontal masonry canopies on either side. Vertical aluminum tubes extended across these masonry slabs. All this created a modern maze of horizontal and vertical elements.

The design was ornate for such a modern building. George Walters recalls that the Southland Center building downtown was constructed just before the Blue Cross building. It was designed in a restrained and minimalist contemporary style. "Someone said it looked like the boxes the Blue Cross building came in," Walters mused.[5]

Though the building was certainly a source of pride to employees, the design did not age well, and, by the early 1980s when the building was on the market (the company having moved to suburban Richardson), one city magazine sarcastically called it downtown's ugliest building.

Whether one considered the building gorgeous or garish, everyone agreed that it was certainly the most posh home the company had ever had, and it announced to the world that Blue Cross and Blue Shield of Texas was big, stable and here to stay.

Inside the building

The interior of the building had 190,966 gross square feet of floor space. Those entering the building were greeted with the message inscribed in the marble along the wall of the elevator bank: "WHAT WE DO FOR OURSELVES DIES WITH US; WHAT WE DO FOR OTHERS REMAINS AND IS IMMORTAL." The quote was a favorite of McBee's and was from Albert Pike, a lawyer turned Episcopal bishop.

In the lobby as throughout the building, marble was used lavishly. Playing as a visual foil against the stately marble in many areas were stark geometric black and white patterns, mirroring McBee's fondness for wearing a white shirt, white tie and black suit.

The first level also contained the reception area where subscribers could come in and discuss claims issues or perhaps pay their dues. McBee made certain that the employees in the reception area were among the company's most personable and cheerful at greeting the public.

Also at ground level and open to the street was a barber shop, placed there by the company as an employee morale builder and also to make the building more attractive to other tenants. The shop never took off. Bourland told McBee, "I had assumed our people would jump at the opportunity of getting their barber work done on company time but apparently a lot of them are still not taking advantage of it."[6] Most likely a lack of other business in that part of downtown—and thus potential clientele—contributed to the poor showing. Bourland also had a difficult time keeping barbers, given the lack of business. By 1962 the company agreed to subsidize the business, but even then it was difficult to make the business a success. The barber shop finally closed in the 1970s.

A public cafeteria was installed on the first floor. It was operated by an outside vendor since the employees' cafeteria on the twelfth floor was subsidized by the company. Floors two through five were reserved for rental in hopes of attracting tenants. However, the company attracted few tenants, for it quickly needed the space for its own expanded operations and had to lease space outside the building within several years.

The building did not follow the usual pattern of having an executive floor with all executives located in a group. Instead, the executive offices were stacked at the northwest corner of the building with one executive on each floor close to the executive's staff. The original locations of top management were:

W. R. McBee, executive director, twelfth floor

Tom Beauchamp, administrative assistant, eleventh floor

R. P. Bourland, director of administration, tenth floor

Medical Director, ninth floor (Lester left in 1959 and was not replaced until 1963 with A. Rex Kirkley, M.D.)

Ralph Webb, director of public relations, eighth floor

Harley B. West, assistant executive director and enrollment director, seventh floor

George Dorsa, comptroller, sixth floor

The seventh floor had conference rooms A and B, which could be combined by moving a partition. The room was designated for enrollment personnel primarily but was also used for THA and TMA meetings. THA itself was housed on the seventh floor. The organization had been headquartered in Dallas and had leased space from the company in the old Blue Cross Building. THA made the move across the street as well, though the organization was in the process of moving to Austin to be closer to the legislative pulse of the state. Ray Hurst was executive director of THA at the time. Conference room C was on the tenth floor.

The twelfth floor employees' cafeteria and lounge were connected by large folding doors. When opened up as one area, 250 people could dine at tables or, when the room was set up as an auditorium, 350 could be seated. The dining room ceiling was two stories tall except at the back of the room where the upper floor was used for storage and a projection booth. One of the more popular features of the building, from the employees' point of view, was the excellent view of the city from the employees' lounge on the twelfth floor. This location was a notable departure from the general practice of putting employees' eating facilities in the basement.

Perhaps the most noticeable feature of the cafeteria was in the ceiling, which featured a suspended cross and shield carved out of the ceiling material. Recessed lighting was placed behind the emblems.

Topping the building was a rotating sign of white porcelain with re-productions of the Blue Cross and Blue Shield service marks, one on each side of the white square. The sign was twenty feet tall and twenty-one feet wide and turned at two revolutions per minute. It had a clutch mechanism which, when the wind velocity reached thirty miles per hour, released the operating mechanism and weathervaned or freed the sign to move parallel with the wind to avoid damage. The lighting was a special neon-type, high-intensity gas. The sign enjoyed unusual visibility be-cause of the building's siting, being the only tall building in that portion of downtown.

With all the exposed symbols of the cross and shield throughout the building, one set of service marks was not seen by most people. On the rooftop, visible only to airplane or helicopter passengers, was a large cross and shield laid in the roof in blue glass chips.

"A working person's utopia"

The technology of the building was space-age current. *Southwest Properties* magazine (a magazine for architects, engineers and real estate people) deemed the building a "working person's utopia."

Although the word "computer" had not yet entered everyday vocabu-lary, the building had several areas with new electronic (it could be said, pre-computer) technology. The RAMAC machine (Random Access Method of Accounting and Control) from IBM was used for billing and reconciliation of direct-pay memberships. This machine abstracted sta-tistical information on group experience and utilization and offered the possibility of later adding equipment for group billing and reconcilia-tion. The Cardatype machines continued to be used to produce member-ship agreements, identification cards and key punch cards. "Robotype" automatic typewriters produced typed letters at 140 words a minute.

The advent of technology was also apparent to employees with the elevators, which were able to operate without an attendant. Marion Trigg, the longtime elevator attendant at the old building, was given the job as guard and greeter in the lobby of the new building. A bank of four Otis Autotronic Elevators whisked employees up and down the twelve stories at five hundred feet per minute. A dumbwaiter also moved mail and records from floor to floor.

The air conditioning system was billed as the most modern available. It used a "double-duct system," which provided a maximum turnover of fresh air. Some of the duct work was outside the building in the alumi-num-clad vertical columns, saving valuable floor space for offices.

It was hoped that the vertical aluminum tubes traversing the horizontal slabs might one day become the vehicles for gathering solar energy that would be piped into the building and then converted to electrical energy. It was an admirable goal that never materialized.

Some of the building's walls were modular. The middle-management and professional offices had moveable walnut-looking metal walls. (The staff was disappointed to discover that the only way to hang pictures was to punch holes in the walls. They were asked not to do this, but eventually the need to hang pictures won out, and the metal walls were punctured.) Noise was also a problem with the metal surface of the panels. Areas with loud equipment had acoustic holes punched in the metal.

Adjoining the building to the north, at the corner of Elm and Central, was a seven-floor parking garage, with each floor of the garage connected to the office building. The garage parked about two hundred cars, and employees were charged ten dollars a month for a space. Though some parking garages of this era relied on attendants to move cars from floor to floor with an elevator, this garage offered ramp access, so employees could park their own cars. There was only a single ramp, however, which proved to be a challenge if a car wanted to exit the garage at the same time another car was entering. Spaces in the garage were somewhat narrow, so drivers were frequently encouraged via memo to be careful and not take up two spaces.

Move-in began in April. Even though the move was just across the street, the company still had to employ movers to load up furniture, drive around the corner and unload in the new space.

The company held a dedication program Wednesday, June 8, 1960, at 11:15 a.m. McBee opened the program, and Sister Mary Helen (board member and administrator of St. Paul Hospital) offered a prayer. Several board members gave remarks. McBee then introduced Dr. W.A. Criswell of First Baptist Church for a brief dedicatory message. The Very Reverend Frank L. Carruthers, dean of St. Matthew's Cathedral (the Episcopal parish that the McBees attended), offered a closing prayer.

As staff settled into their shiny new home, they were getting ready for a major new piece of business.

During the summer of 1959, President Dwight Eisenhower signed the Federal Employees Health Benefits Program into law, to take effect on July 1, 1960. It was a major opportunity for Blue Cross and Blue Shield Plans, but, since it was a national program, it would require high levels of cooperation and coordination in the System.

The Texas Plan was already experienced in working with federal employees. For years, the Plan had enrolled many post offices, several military bases and the Red River Arsenal in Texarkana. All of these groups had been sold individually, premiums were collected with no payroll deduction and employers had not contributed to the cost of the coverage.

The legislation provided for a standard national program under the supervision of the Civil Service Commission. Blue Cross and Blue Shield Plans and commercial carriers from a syndicate headed by Aetna were invited to participate. Under the provisions of the legislation, each carrier would offer two types of plans with a high and low level of benefits, and the government would contribute toward the cost of coverage. Federal employees would have the choice of these various plans.

Carriers could work out rate and benefit information and had to do so quickly. In the case of the Blue System, the Blue Cross Association and the National Association of Blue Shield Plans would bid as prime contractors and would subcontract with Plans. For the first time in the System's history, the Plans presented a united front. The size of the potential enrollment probably helped Plans to put aside their differences.

The Texas Plan scampered to establish rates and benefits in line with the government requirements and began to enroll federal employees. Training for hospitals was implemented. Four teams of staff spanned the state to host workshops for hospitals on how to handle the new volume of federal employee business. By the end of the year, McBee reported to the board that the company had received good cooperation from the hospitals. Enrollment of federal employees and dependents stood at approximately 150,000, more than half of the business in Texas.

But a problem remained. The Civil Service Commission required experience rating on the medical-surgical side of coverage. Because of state laws, GM&SS, as a mutual insurance company, could not experience rate. The basic point in Texas law was that each GM&SS member should receive the same consideration as any other member, so experience rating would discriminate among members. Again, the limitations of GM&SS being a mutual company were apparent.

The board authorized a study to determine if GM&SS should be converted into a legal reserve company. At first the board approved the conversion but then determined a better course of action that would to allow the company greater flexibility in underwriting. They decided to buy a stock company that could do what needed to be done. McBee announced to the board that the stock of the American Savings Life Insurance Company of Houston was for sale.

Not only would this give the company the flexibility to meet the demands for the new Federal Employee Program, it would allow the company's entry into yet another important market—life insurance. For years the company had partnered with a life insurance company to offer package benefits to a group, an arrangement that was often less than satisfactory.

This third company operated under the familiar cross and shield service marks; its name was changed to Group Life and Health Insurance Company and the home office was moved from Houston to Dallas. The new corporation could write whatever was needed on the medical-surgical side, even hospitalization if desired. It could own a home office building and sell life, accident and disability insurance.

The board approved the transaction on August 12, 1960, and the sale was completed by December. Board president L. H. Allen was made president of GLH, and McBee served in the combined offices of vice president-secretary-treasurer. (GLH had an interlocking board of directors with GHS and GM&SS, similar to that of GM&SS.) An October 5, 1960, memo to all employees from McBee announced the purchase. The company's first piece of business was to issue accident insurance to employees.

The first group life insurance case written was effective May 1, 1961. The business of life insurance, of course, was new to the company and sent the staff into a flurry of activity to make sense of the new world. As McBee told Beauchamp, "Our object is to GET GOING and get going in all directions. We want Action!"[7]

Beauchamp, with his former experience at the state board of insurance, provided much counsel. The addition of GLH also required more sophisticated financial managers in the company. McBee hired Walter F. Hachmeister from the Blue Cross Association (BCA), who began July 1, 1961. Hired as assistant comptroller, Hachmeister had a strong finance background and much of it with a commercial insurer. He had been with Kemper Insurance Company from 1950 to 1959 and then took a job with the Blue Cross Commission, which was shortly merged into the BCA. Hachmeister's commercial experience was attractive to McBee, faced as he was with putting together a life insurance company.

Plenty of new activities were required to set up the life insurance company: products had to be designed, rates set and policy forms established. Especially pressing was the question of whether to move business from GM&SS and, if so, how and when. Since GLH was a stock company, taxes were an issue. In addition, decisions had to be made about which of these issues existing staff could handle and who should be hired to handle the rest.

The Texas Plan was the first in the nation to purchase or form its own life insurance company. This caused some consternation among the Plans that going into the life insurance business was not a wise move. However, eventually many other Plans followed Texas' lead and began to purchase or form life insurance companies.

By the end of 1961, twenty life groups were enrolled, individual policies were sold and the monthly rate of premium income on life business was approaching $4,000 with a combined monthly premium of about $112,000. At the end of the first three years of operation, the company had about $65 million of life insurance in force. GLH went on to be licensed in several states, serving Blue Cross Plans as their life affiliate and becoming a very successful business. In early 1963 a Blue Shield license was granted to GLH, so the new company began taking on more of the medical-surgical business. Gradually, business was transferred from GM&SS to GLH.

After the watershed year of 1960 and by the beginning of 1961, it was obvious that much was changing for the company. Membership was growing. When the company first occupied its leased space in October 1946, Blue Cross membership stood at a little more than 195,000 and Blue Shield membership had just started. By the end of 1960, the Texas Plan led all Plans in new enrollments (136,390 new Blue Cross memberships and 113,324 Blue Shield memberships). Now, memberships in both Blue Cross and Blue Shield hovered at around 1.3 million. A new third corporation gave the Texas Plan new flexibility in meeting market demand. A major new account with the Federal Employee Program afforded the company important experience in working with the federal government.

But as significant as 1960 had been and as much change as it had brought, even greater changes, challenges and opportunities were just around the corner.

9 | 1961-1967: Exponential Growth

> *"All in all, this is going to be about the most*
> *eventful year in our history."*
> *Walter R. McBee*

By the early 1960s, speculation was occurring again about the need for government-sponsored health care for underserved segments of the population. The plight of the elderly was the primary concern, but the indigent population was also the subject of ongoing discussion.

The subject was being discussed in the company board room. Early in the decade, the company's position on government involvement in health care was essentially divided. On the one hand, the company's heritage had been one of service to society, of helping people help themselves, and the company showed a natural interest in the plight of the elderly. On the other hand, McBee as well as the board were deeply distrustful of government's role in health care. The company's history had proven the validity of the "voluntary principle," that the private sector could help solve societal problems.

As early as October 1959, the company mounted an assertive individual enrollment campaign by mail to demonstrate that private enterprise could help societal problems. During October only, any Texan aged sixty-five and older could apply for an individual policy. The campaign enrolled 5,797 subscribers over age sixty-five (as well as 3,113 under sixty-five). The campaign demonstrated the company's intention to serve the senior population, but it was hardly an outstanding success. One difficulty in getting seniors to enroll was that many of them were waiting to see what would happen with the federal legislation everyone was talking about.

Changes in the Social Security Act (voted in 1956, 1958 and 1960) had increased federal participation in helping states provide funds for indigent health care. The 1960 law included a special plan for the aged who were medically needy and not on public assistance. It set up a matching grant program with the federal government paying from 50 to 80 percent of the costs. There had been talk of a federal program for the elderly that would be financed through Social Security and would be available to all senior citizens, regardless of income.

While the company resisted federal involvement in health care, it took interest in this federal- and state-financed Old Age Assistance Program (OAA), made possible by the Kerr-Mills amendment in the Social Security law.

In September 1961 McBee outlined the details of the program to the board, explaining that 220,000 recipients were on the rolls and that the company would get twelve dollars a month per recipient to insure them.

Unlike the specter of using Social Security funds to pay for health care for the aged, the AMA and AHA supported the OAA program thoroughly.

The board authorized staff to proceed with negotiations. The company issued a bid that projected a mere 3 percent for administrative overhead but not without concern among officers that costs might exceed that amount.

Statistician Annie Laurie Surratt expressed a lack of confidence in the rates the company was proposing. Beauchamp agreed that the business would certainly add gloss to the company's roster of enrolled groups, "but can we afford the prestige?" he quizzed McBee.[1]

Despite the concerns, the company went ahead with the bid and was told in August that it was the selected vendor. With the program startup of January 1, 1962, the company had barely 130 days to get ready for 220,000 new members—the largest group ever enrolled by the company.

It was a Texas-sized task with very little time available to accomplish it. Especially pressing was the need for more automated processing of claims. The company had a data processing department since the 1940s, but the technology of the era went no further than making punch cards. A clerk sat at a large tab-impact machine and punched information into cards that were used for billings, membership information and automated correspondence. This technology, though it speeded many clerical tasks, couldn't process information or "think."

It was the next generation of data processing that introduced the actual computer. Gene Aune, then manager of the Case Department, recalled that computers were just beginning to come off the assembly lines. McBee had promised the welfare department that the company would get a computer. "We didn't know a computer from a garbage can. We immediately scrambled around and, of course, we had all IBM punch card equipment so obviously we called IBM."[2]

The account executive at IBM was a 31-year-old salesman named Ross Perot.

The company's first computer

The company also called another computer manufacturer and was seriously considering buying from this competitor. But Perot got the sale since he could also procure programmers for the new computer, something the other company couldn't do.

In those early days of computing, supply couldn't keep up with demand, and companies often had to wait to get their new computers. However, Blue Cross and Blue Shield of Texas couldn't wait—the clock was ticking, and it had to get up and running.

Perot demonstrated to his new client exactly how aggressive and smart he was. He found a provision in the law stating that if substantial change in legislation had occurred, a customer could get a needed computer without waiting in line. The enabling legislation had in fact been recently revised in June 1961, so IBM approved Perot's request to go to the head of the line for the computer.

Around Thanksgiving IBM began delivering the equipment—an IBM 1401 computer. The 1401 consisted of several units, including a main processing unit with a punch card feeder (punch cards fed data into the machine, which then translated the data to tape) and a printer. It was thought to be the second such computer in Dallas, and now that it was delivered, the question was what to do with it.

Two of Aune's employees from the Case Department, Jack Buzbee and Jack Davis, were loaned to work with Perot. Buzbee was sent to IBM computer school and learned computer programming. Perot also brought in several men who knew how to program computers.

Aune and the staff would tell the computer experts what they needed from the computer. "We would sit with them and explain," Aune recalled. "They didn't know what we were talking about and we didn't know what they were talking about. But we explained the kind of records we needed to keep, that we needed access to update it, that we had to keep track of limitations and exclusions and so forth and so on. They would run stuff and bring it back to us and we'd look at it and we'd tweak it here and there, and they'd go back and fix it."[3]

Buzbee recalled the long days and nights. "We worked 18 hours a day. We worked from early in the morning to 10 at night, for six or seven days a week and for two or three months. We were isolated from the rest of the company. We all were in one room with the machinery and maybe a couple or three desks."[4]

While the company was gearing up for the business, the contract with the state was signed November 15, "with all the ceremonies of a regimental dress parade," Beauchamp ruminated.[5]

Radio spots purchased by the company touted the Texas Plan's strength: "Another FIRST for TEXAS! Another FIRST for BLUE CROSS! But BLUE CROSS is ALWAYS first!" And the ad ended with a chorus singing, "In all the hospital-medical field, there's NOTHING like BLUE CROSS-BLUE SHIELD!"[6]

Despite the hype of the radio ad, it was authentically an historic moment. Though several Blue Cross and Blue Shield Plans ended up administering OAA programs in their territories, the Texas Plan was the first to be involved in the program. And Texas was a significant state given the size of its population eligible for OAA.

Newspapers across the state reported on the event. The banner headline of *The Houston Press* captured best the feeling about the event: "Texas Makes History."

The initial contract for the OAA program ran from January 1, 1962 to August 31, 1963. Fred Rodgers managed the program. Ken Patteson had been hired into the management trainee program in 1963 and in 1964 was made a supervisor of the OAA program in the Case Department.

In the program, a qualified recipient received a certificate that would be recognized at a hospital for a physician-ordered hospitalization. The program was financed by state funds (25 percent) and federal funds (75 percent), with the state controlling the program. The program also included some nursing home benefits, which were administered separately from the hospitalization. Blue Cross and Blue Shield of Texas got $8.68 a month per recipient in exchange for providing hospital care.

On the first business day of January 1962, staff pushed the "On" button, and the company's first real computer went to work.

The computer worked as hoped, and the program was successful from every other angle as well. The company had entered the transaction holding its corporate breath, but it was an astounding success. The first case was received and processed on January 3, and within a few months the company was processing about seven thousand cases each month.

After just a couple of months of operation, McBee told the board that the OAA program had operated more smoothly than expected. By the end of the year, he reported that not only had implementation been successful but also the utilization of benefits had amounted to less than 90 percent of premiums. This meant that the cost of operating the OAA program had amounted to just under the allowance of 3 percent of premiums. The contract was renewed in September 1963 for two years. At one point the company returned one million dollars to the state that had been earned in investments off of the money made.

One of the most noticeable effects of the OAA within the company was how it catapulted the company into the future of data processing. Once the OAA program was up and running and the company understood how to use the new computer technology, staff began a systematic conversion of virtually all systems to computers. Buzbee recalled that the group billing system was converted to a computer file, a process that consumed about a year. Next, the direct pay files were converted, and eventually the claims system also entered the electronic era. The department that had been staffed by two employees, a vendor and a handful of outside experts mushroomed into a staff of 100 people. On August 1, 1962, Ross Perot was hired away from IBM as the manager of the Advanced Systems and Development Department. He said he had become dissatisfied with IBM's limits on sales quotas.

Perot, however, was to work at Blue Cross and Blue Shield of Texas only half time. The other half was used in setting up his own company: Electronic Data Systems (EDS). It was an unusual relationship but gave the company the advantage of attracting and retaining sophisticated systems engineers for a business that was becoming ever more sophisticated. It also benefited Perot by giving him an income as he set up his own company. Perot's office was located on the sixth floor, and he reported to Hahn. He was an employee until November 30, 1967, when he moved EDS to a location in Exchange Park in Dallas.

Changes in the company

As the company moved into the modern era of computers, it was affected by world events far away from Dallas and Texas.

The Cuban missile crisis, which held a nation in suspense, began to affect company operations. Harley West took a military leave of absence in October 1961 to take command as major general of the 49th Armored Division in Fort Polk, Louisiana. (Several other men left on military leave as well.) He returned to his post the next year and in a short memo to staff on August 17 gleefully announced, "I am back! I am real glad to be back! I am at the office! Let's all go to work!"[7]

Meanwhile, the local civil defense commission worked with downtown businesses to create fallout shelters in case of a nuclear strike on downtown Dallas. Only the basements of the Blue Cross Building and the attached garage qualified as fallout shelters. The company participated, putting up the familiar fallout shelter signs, and at least one person was sent to fallout manager's school.

By the early 1960s, Blue Cross and Blue Shield coverage was considered the Cadillac of medical insurance. The 1962 edition of *Webster's New World Dictionary* even contained a definition of Blue Cross, so the name had become a household word. Despite the premier status of the Blue Cross and Blue Shield brand name, it was clear that commercial competition and an increasingly sophisticated consumer market would require the company to continue to improve operations and marketing to advance its position.

An executive planning committee of Bourland, Beauchamp, Hachmeister and Higginbotham was formed that made a sweeping list of suggestions in a 1963 document titled *Ten Points for Progress*. The document identified problems and solutions. The preface asked, "How far have we come since our organization first started back in 1939?" The committee looked at the answers and decided that the company needed several major changes in order to advance in the demanding and competitive market.

Foremost was a hard push for more sales. Several sales contests were instituted. The 1962 "Top Gun" contest offered a catalog of prizes for sales personnel and ended with the awards given by executives adorned in western wear, six-shooters included. Even the dignified McBee dressed in costume. More prestigious was the "Executive Director's Award" introduced to honor the top salesman for 1963. Duke Landry was its first recipient.

A Market Research Department started in 1963 with Ralph Webb as manager. In June 1963 the company made a move to bring the language of the company in line with the commercial insurance industry—the Service Department was renamed the Underwriting Department. The newly named department put all the company's underwriting functions, including GL&H, in one department. Don Spradley was named manager of the new section.

In September 1963 a glossy company publication premiered: *Quota Busters*. It was a four-page publication dedicated to honoring top sales leaders and contained sales tips and news of the enrollment area. The cover of each issue featured Bob Kimbrell's famous pencil portrait illustrations. The first issue's Man of the Month was Charles Brock of the Fort Worth sales office. Austin sales representative Francis Bolton was the first female Man of the Month in January 1965. On the cover of that issue, "Man" was shown with a slash through it, and the word "Woman" inserted above it.

In October 1965 Jerry Thompson was named to fill the new position of director of sales promotion concurrently with his position as a regional sales director. In the announcement memo, Enrollment Director West said, "We are gearing for action—more action—positive action—motivated by and designed with a determination for bigger and better results...."[8]

As part of this gearing up for new action, Blue Cross was continually improving coverage. In October 1960 the company introduced a special Educator's Service and expanded it in 1962 to allow small groups of ten to twenty-five members to enroll. In 1961 the Supplemental Catastrophic Illness Endorsement was introduced with some expanded benefits. (As an indication of where medical technology stood, the coverage still listed the iron lung as a benefit.)

In June 1961 the company introduced major medical supplemental coverages.

In 1965 the company premiered a major new product that was to stay on the market for many years. Before 1965 only standard health care coverage plans were offered, with employers choosing from a preset menu. Benefits were varied only in competitive situations based on the size of the group. Custom Coverage was introduced to give groups new flexibility in benefit combinations. The addition of this one product meant that employer groups suddenly had an array of choices in health care coverage. Custom Coverage offered a building block design, allowing the group to select provisions of the policy, such as room and board allowance, maximum days of hospital confinement and level of surgical benefits.

A more aggressive sales operation needed a more aggressive communications program. A flashing sign was added at the top of the north side of the building (facing North Central Expressway) in 1965. It was 113 feet wide, 8 ½ feet tall and commanded an audience of 120,000 viewers daily from the expressway. A series of ten different panels flashed messages such as "Welcome to Dallas, City of Excellence," or "Welcome to Dallas, Birthplace of Blue Cross." The sign would occasionally give health or safety tips ("Seat Belts Save Lives") or welcome a visiting dignitary by name.

All of this activity paid off in 1966 when the company celebrated yet another milestone—membership reached and then surpassed two million participants.

Despite the marketplace successes of the decade, the company was increasingly concerned about the cost of health care, which seemed to be rising constantly. The company had ceased to be a financing arm for the hospitals and now, incrementally, was beginning to become a separate force on health care costs and delivery.

In response to cost pressures, in 1964 the group experience rating system was replaced by one that applied rate increases to groups on their anniversary dates. The formula used both the group's experience and community rating. The larger the group, the more the rate was tied to its utilization; the smaller the group, the more the rate relied on combined community experience. By the end of 1965, even this had to be updated with faster and higher increases to keep pace.

The presidency of the board changed several times during the decade. Board president L. H. Allen died on August 24, 1964. E. A. Rowley, M.D., took the reins of the position until April 10, 1965, when James W. Aston was installed. John Justin, Jr., who became chairman of the board in 1979 after Aston's term, was elected to the board at the March 1963 meeting.

Assistant Comptroller Walter F. Hachmeister became comptroller in 1965.

At the March board meeting in 1967, the board, in a move to bring the company more into the mainstream of business, approved a bylaws amendment that changed several titles in the company. The executive director became president and the president of the board became chairman of the board. The title change became effective in April. At the same time, Beauchamp was made assistant secretary and Hachmeister, assistant treasurer. Several years earlier Beauchamp's staff title had changed from administrative assistant, which no longer really described his job, to legal counsel.

Medical Director A. Rex Kirkley accepted the position of manager of the Washington, D.C., office of the AMA in April 1967, and Doyle W. Ferguson, M.D., was named medical director.

Opposition to federal financing

Though the OAA program was a huge success in Texas, such was not true everywhere else. States were uneven in the way they handled the program. Despite the advances of OAA in some localities, people were still talking about a purely federally financed program for the aged and one that would be available to all senior citizens, not means tested. In February 1961 President John F. Kennedy called for a program that would provide hospital and nursing home coverage for all Americans over age sixty-five, financed by an increase in Social Security taxes. A few days later, the King-Anderson bills were introduced in Congress, and the debate was on.

At first both the AMA and AHA stood firm against further federal legislation. Many Plan leaders did also, fearing that the King-Anderson initiative represented a severe encroachment on the voluntary basis of health care. McBee was among these Plan leaders, and the board was behind him. Even with the successes of handling OAA and the Federal Employee Program (FEP), company leaders remained wary about the federal financing of medical care for the aged. In the OAA program, control stayed at the local level, even though federal dollars financed three-fourths of the program.

At the board meeting of Sept. 15, 1961, the members passed a resolution in support of the "American way of life and voluntary prepayment of health insurance" and opposed to "federally controlled and financed programs of health care." The resolution indicated that the federal legislative proposals to provide health care to the aged through the Social Security system would "stymie the growth of voluntary health insurance and ultimately lead to its decline."

Walter McNerney, the new president of the BCA, urged the Plans to stay flexible. It was becoming clear that the Plans could be in a good position to act as intermediaries if the legislation ever became reality.

To further demonstrate how Texas could solve its own problems, the company introduced Senior Texan Service in March 1962. It was an extension and refinement of the 1959 individual enrollment. It provided hospitalization and medical-surgical protection as well as limited nursing home care.

By 1963 the Texas Plan was well involved with federal programs. The OAA and FEP programs accounted for a significant percentage of Plan enrollment and operations.

A turnabout on Medicare

It became clearer that not only *could* the company become an intermediary but that it *should,* since it (as well as Plans across the nation) had the experience and expertise to administer the program effectively on behalf of the public. The board dropped official opposition to the concept by 1965 when they agreed that should the company be called upon to act as the intermediary administrative agency, "the Texas Plan will do its usual outstanding job and that its aim will always be to give its members the best possible service at the lowest possible cost."[9]

By the time President Lyndon B. Johnson signed the historic bill that created Medicare on July 30, 1965, the program had evolved into three programs. Title 18 of the Social Security Act was split into two programs. Medicare Part A offered hospital, nursing home and home health services. Medicare Part B provided benefits for physician care. Part A was compulsory, while Part B was voluntary. The act also consisted of Title

19, which provided Medicaid health care benefits for the indigent under age sixty-five. The Medicare program went into effect on July 1, 1966.

With the signing of the legislation, the Texas Plan again had only a few months to prepare for a huge increase in responsibilities—and the beginning of a new era in public-private partnership. Under the act, hospitals could nominate the intermediaries for Part A. Blue Cross Plans were selected as intermediaries in thirty-one states. The BCA acted as a prime contractor for Part A and then subcontracted with the Plans. Under Part B, the intermediaries were called carriers and were appointed by the secretary of the federal Department of Health, Education and Welfare. GHS was the Part A intermediary, and GM&SS assumed the role as Part B carrier. (GM&SS no longer was the primary Blue Shield company. In 1963 the Blue Shield license also was granted to Group Life and Health Insurance Company.)

McBee noted the new reality facing the company:

> The responsibility that confronts us in acting as intermediary for both Parts A (hospital claims) and B (physician claims) of Medicare is a very imposing one. It involves a lot of "tooling up," including recruitment of something like 165 to 175 additional employees, as well as all of the working equipment. More than that, it entails coming to grips with a vast array of new laws, regulations, procedures and personalities. I have no concern about our ability to perform, but neither am I unaware of the fact we are going to have our hands full for a while.
>
> All in all, this is going to be about the most eventful year in our history. It is a difficult but challenging outlook. With all of the new things coming at us at once, it would be easy for our people to become distracted from the pursuit of those that constitute our basic reason for existence, but we are not going to be led astray; and I already feel a certain amount of pride about the accomplishments and report we will be bringing to you a year from today.[10]

Even though McBee had initial misgivings about government involvement in Medicare, he approached the program pragmatically. Beauchamp recalled that his attitude was, "All right, it is the law. We lost that battle. Now, we can stand off and continue to spit at it or we can say, since this is going to be done...we want to get in on the action."[11]

There was much to do to prepare for the program. In April 1966 a group of about twenty-five people were hired to handle claims. In May and June a team of executives conducted workshops across the state for hospitals and doctors in a whirlwind series of twenty-one meetings in thirteen days, beginning in Tyler and ending in Wichita Falls.

The Senior Texan Service had to be redesigned to complement Medicare benefits and became the Senior Texan Companion Service, offered in two tiers of benefit coverage: basic and major medical.

Company managers and field staff had to become familiar with Medicare benefits. Field staff had to contact virtually every group to modify benefits for employees or retirees who were sixty-five years or older. Those over sixty-five could transfer their coverage to Medicare, supplemented by the Senior Texan Companion Service.

Frank Henry was the first manager of Medicare, with Fred Higginbotham providing executive leadership. (Higginbotham had been hired in 1961 and gradually assumed leadership of both public and professional relations. He eventually left the Texas Plan to become president of the Plan in Atlanta, Georgia.)

A second group of more than twenty employees was hired in June. Barbara Harvey was one of those employees. Hired as a Medicare claims examiner, years later she became a vice president of the subsidiary corporation established for Medicare. She recalled that on July 1 she and the others sat around waiting for claims. At first, they received no claims. Then, they began to trickle in. "When the first ones came in, we passed them around and discussed what code we should put on each claim," she recalled. About a month later, however, the troupe didn't have time for academic discussions of which codes to use. "They started coming in and never stopped," Harvey recalled. "We were overwhelmed with the volume. The claims system was not automated as it is today. We coded the claim on the claim form itself or we actually used a coding transcript, a form where we put information and the claims were passed over to the keypunch people. It was very, very manually oriented."

Initially, Harvey said, the room was awash in paper claims. "The thing that I remember the most is claims weren't put into batches. They came up on the dumbwaiter and we had four control clerks and they passed claims out. Everybody just had stacks of individual claims on their desks."

In those early days, the processes were incredibly simple as compared to the program's later computer-tight efficiency. "If someone called in to check on a claim, the supervisor would just say, 'Please go through your claims; do you have Mrs. Smith's?'" At the end of the day staff would count claims to determine the number that were pending. One supervisor, Harvey recalled, got smart and had the examiners measure claims instead of counting them, arriving at a formula that an inch equaled so many claims. If an examiner had a question about coding, the supervisor would sometimes use a megaphone to give the answer.

The public didn't uniformly understand the new program, Harvey says. "There was a lot of confusion with the public on what Medicare was. We got claims with all sorts of bills, not just health care bills. We had one claim where the beneficiary had attached her electric bill, an airplane ticket and household bills like that. She thought that Medicare would pay all her bills during her illness!"

By December it was clear that the staff couldn't handle the unexpected initial volume. Employees throughout the company were asked to pitch in to help pay claims. They worked their regular jobs during the day, had dinner in the employees' cafeteria and then worked four more hours on Medicare. "We had everyone working, including the executive director's secretary and people from Engineering," Harvey said. "Those of us who were supposed to know what we were doing walked around answering questions. Our coding manual was about the size of a steno notepad. We didn't have lots of codes in those days."[12]

The keypunch people were similarly overwhelmed. Lelia Fischer (later Wright) was a keypunch operator in the company, hired in 1957. She was transferred to the new Medicare department and eventually became a senior vice president of government programs. She remembered there were "key shops" around the city which served businesses by punching data cards. "We went to key shops all over town, hired people, taught them how to keypunch, as well as having our own classes," Wright recalled. "While many employees were recruited to work extra hours for Medicare, the keypunch operators had a particularly demanding schedule. We worked ten hours on and then we were off five hours, then back on ten hours, for seven days a week for a period of time, trying to train these people and get it up and running."[13]

Early in 1967 Medicare employees moved from the Blue Cross Building into leased space downtown. Claims staff went to the Hartford Building, and keypunch personnel went to the Dallas Federal building. The earlier hopes of leasing out several floors of the home office building were dashed by the incredible growth in the company. By the mid-1960s, the building was full.

By early 1968 the chaos had settled into an efficient process.

With the advent of Medicare, the company's budget and employees mushroomed. In 1961 the company processed a little more than $55 million in total benefit payments. In the first eighteen months of the Medicare program (July 1966 through December 1967), the company paid combined Parts A and B Medicare benefits of $234 million. Regular business benefits for the full year of 1967 were over $128 million. To handle this increased activity, the employee population had grown to more than fifteen hundred.

It was clear that after Medicare, both the company and the health care industry had changed. McBee described this new era in a speech to the THA: "The final curtain has fallen on the era of 'horse-and-buggy' medical practice and kitchen table surgery, it's fallen on the 'house of mystery' type operation of the hospital, and it's fallen on the 'haphazard' marketing and administration of prepaid health care protection. The overture is being played, however, and the curtain is rising on a new era."[14]

Part of that new era was the Medicaid program for indigent Americans, created by the same federal legislation that created Medicare.

Medicare essentially put the OAA program out of business, since Medicare provided coverage for all Americans over the age of sixty-five, including those who had been on OAA rolls. The state, which was already funding OAA, realized that with the savings afforded by Medicare, they could expand the rolls and offer health coverage to other welfare recipients, the blind, disabled and dependent children. The program also paid the Medicare coinsurance and deductible for aged welfare recipients.

As a result, the OAA program ended in June 1966 after four and one-half years of highly successful administration by the Texas Plan. During that time the Texas Plan had paid more than $100 million in benefits and served a population of up to 228,000 Texans.

In July the program was expanded to include the blind, disabled and dependent children and called simply the Kerr-Mills Program after the legislation that had fathered the original OAA program. It provided funds to help senior citizens pay their Medicare coinsurance and deductible amounts. The company signed a contract with the state to administer the new program.

A year later, Medicaid put that program out of business. Title 19 of the Social Security act, or Medicaid, became effective in Texas on September 1, 1967, and supplanted the Kerr-Mills program. Medicaid served more than 351,000 recipients. According to law, Medicaid intermediaries were chosen by the states. In Texas, the company was chosen as the Medicaid intermediary. It was, in fact, the first in the nation to administer Medicaid on an underwritten basis. In other states, intermediaries often just served an administrative function.

Twilight of an era

In 1967 renowned Dallas artist Dmitri Vail was commissioned to paint McBee's portrait. Vail's résumé of subjects included many notable figures of the day, including Presidents John Kennedy and Lyndon Johnson and many entertainment celebrities. In a special ceremony, Lillian McBee unveiled the portrait, and it was given to the employees of the company, to be hung in the hallway outside the twelfth-floor executive offices. (Today, it hangs on the second floor east entry to the main building in Richardson.)

As the year progressed, McBee's vibrancy began to dim. On one trip to Amarillo, he exited the plane and couldn't remember which city he was in. Several times in the home office building, he would leave to go downtown and then return to quizzically ask his secretary, "Where was I going?"

The memory lapses grew worse, and in August he went to the doctor and was admitted to the hospital for tests. The diagnosis was a brain tumor, and he was scheduled immediately for surgery, which he underwent on August 28. A special session of the executive committee met on that day and appointed Tom Beauchamp as interim chief executive officer during McBee's expected recuperation. A memo to employees said McBee might be recuperating for thirty days.

Unfortunately, he never awoke from the operation and died on August 30. He was only sixty-four years old. The news of his death, perhaps not completely unexpected given the severity of his illness, nonetheless threw the company into shock. "Nobody knew the company could be run by anyone except him," Aune said. "It was an uncertain time."[15]

Funeral services were held on September 1 at St. Matthews Episcopal Cathedral, with interment at Restland Memorial Park in North Dallas. All Blue Cross and Blue Shield of Texas offices closed in his memory on that day.

In some newspaper obituaries McBee was called "the Father of Blue Cross." Interestingly, that was the same title bestowed on Justin Ford Kimball in some obituaries eleven years earlier. It can be said that Blue Cross in Texas had two fathers: Kimball began the concept; McBee gave the company a successful life after a very shaky start.

McBee had joined a new company struggling not only to thrive as an organization, but also as an idea. Could the financing of hospital costs through a voluntary prepayment plan succeed? He had brought his stately bearing and his strong beliefs in free enterprise to build a lasting institution. By 1967 the environment was more complex, with government assuming a new role in health care, the company becoming more competitive in its regular business and cost increases severely pressuring the whole health care system. It was a different entity altogether than the one he had come to salvage in 1941.

During McBee's twenty-six year tenure, the company had grown from a small operation in a little building of twenty-seven employees to a mature giant of the industry, employing 1,503 employees in its gleaming twelve-story skyscraper. Membership had grown from seventy-five thousand in 1941 to more than two million in 1967. The life company had more than $617 million of insurance in force, and the company was successfully administering several government health care programs.

McBee's accomplishments didn't stop at the company. He was known across the nation of Blue Cross and Blue Shield Plans; was a member of the board of governors of the BCA, since its formation in 1960; was a member of the executive committee and treasurer of the Blue Cross Commission; served two terms as Blue Shield Commissioner of District IX region and was an advisor to the AMA's insurance committee. A lifetime member of the THA and Northwest Texas Hospital Association, he was an associate member of the Southern Medical Association.

He was known among the powerful leaders of Dallas and was a member of the Dallas Citizens Council, Greater Dallas Planning Commission, Trinity Improvement Association, Citizens Traffic Commission, Dallas Chamber of Commerce, Texas Police Association, Texas Association of Life Insurance Officials, Texas Association of Manufacturers and the U.S. Chamber of Commerce. He served on the boards of the Central Business District Association of Dallas and the Dallas Civic Opera. Governor John Connally had appointed him to the Commission on Aging.

In his religious life he was senior warden of St. Matthew's Cathedral and chaired many committees and causes for improvement in the parish.

Adding to his legacy is the people he hired, nurtured and treated, in the final analysis, as his family. He was a patriarch, in the best sense of the word.

Aune recalled him this way:

> McBee very thoroughly enjoyed having a company party where his "family" was there. Keep in mind he and Lillian had no family and no kids, but he could get all the executives and department managers and their wives or husbands or girlfriends or boyfriends and we would just have a morning brunch or a dinner party. That's when he was the father figure and he loved it. He cared about people.

> You respected him because the man would walk in and here's this beautifully dressed man with this flowing hair. You knew he was in the room. He had presence. Men and women paid attention. I thought it was great to have a boss so distinguished looking. People would ask, "Who's your boss?" and you were proud to answer, "Walter McBee!"[16]

In the days that followed his sudden death, everyone looked around to see who could replace the fallen giant. It seemed impossible that anyone but Walter R. McBee could lead Blue Cross and Blue Shield of Texas.

10 | 1968-1979: The Challenges of Change

"The spirit that I read in the top echelons of our organization these days could well be expressed as a slogan, borrowing that famous line, 'The past is prologue.' A free translation of that is, 'You ain't seen nothin' yet!'"
Tom L. Beauchamp

Employees returned to work on Tuesday, September 5, 1967. With the Labor Day holiday on Monday, it had been four days since the company had been open. Things were different, however. The man who had rescued the company and built it into a formidable force in the industry was gone.

Beauchamp continued in the role of acting president. In March 1968 the board unanimously elected him president.

McBee and Beauchamp certainly had different styles of leadership. Whereas McBee could be said to have been captain of the ship during his tenure, Beauchamp became more of the guardian of the company. McBee's style was dashing, and his presence filled the room, while Beauchamp was down to earth, shy, methodical, deliberate, quiet and concerned with details.

Tom L. Beauchamp, Jr., was born December 16, 1913, in Paris, Texas. He married his high school sweetheart, Eleanor Aden, known as Honey. After receiving a bachelor's and a law degree from the University of Texas at Austin, he practiced law in Tyler from 1938 to 1939. From 1939 to 1940 he served as assistant state auditor and the next year became secretary to the Texas governor (serving briefly both W. Lee O'Daniel and Coke Stevenson). After a year in this capacity, he became an examiner for the

Texas Insurance Department where as an apprentice he was assigned to work with the struggling Group Hospital Service. McBee hired him in 1944. He became very active in civic affairs and served one term on the Dallas City Council. He was a layman at the White Rock Methodist Church, and active in the Kiwanis Club and the Circle Ten Council of the Boy Scouts. He and Honey had one son, Tom Beauchamp III.

As a lawyer Beauchamp brought great attention to detail in his work for the company. He studied any proposal from a number of angles and insisted on having a plan. He was the company philosopher as well as its leader. His earlier positions with the company were diverse and his job responsibilities broad. He served as office manager, administrative assistant, purchasing agent, forms designer and legal counsel.

But his role as president was well defined, and he entered the job focused on leading the company forward and moving it into the modern world of corporations. Clearly, McBee had been a patriarch—he loved the company and loved its people. But the world of business was growing beyond the scope of patriarchy. Blue Cross and Blue Shield of Texas was now the holder of several major and important government contracts. The company had to mature, and it was Beauchamp who would move the company into an era of modern management principles.

He began by formulating a master plan. In early January Beauchamp attended an American Management Association seminar and decided that management should have the benefit of the association's Top Management Briefings. He sent executive staff to the briefings, and they were enthusiastic about the information they received. As a result of the briefings, the company held two-day retreats with the purpose of formulating a long-range planning program.

The result was published later in 1968 as *The Challenge and the Plan*, covering the period from November 1, 1968, to December 31, 1971. It was the company's first corporate plan, an attempt to formalize company goals and procedures and move the company to a full corporate structure. In the foreword, Beauchamp emphasized the necessity of the company being a progressive operation.

> In the field of health care, the pace of evolution is now so rapid that it might more properly be characterized as "revolution." Correspondingly, new concepts related to the role, scope and methodology of prepayment are emerging constantly. Recognizing these "facts of life," we have—individually and as a team—taken inventory of our present position. We have catalogued and evaluated our strengths, our deficiencies and our opportunities...As the result, we have agreed upon this Corporate Plan and pledge our dedication to its fulfillment.

The booklet translated the challenges of the modern market into corporate objectives: Increase market share by the addition of 272,000 members; increase life products in force; improve relationships with health care providers; enhance the public image of the company; increase surplus or reserves to protect members; increase efficiency and reduce cost, and become even more active in regional (District IX) and national issues.

Meeting the challenge

The company developed new departments, new processes and new ways of thinking to meet the challenges of the late 1960s and early 1970s. The company's advertising took a more positive approach. "Join the Big Parade" shouted the headline, and then in blue ink a subhead reminded the reader, "the swing is to the 'blues'!" The ad positioned the company's stability and longevity in the business with the verve of the emerging youth culture.

By 1968 "Enrollment Representatives" had become "Sales Representatives." "'Sales' is a more appropriate term," said West, "because it carries a connotation of selling some business."[1] The traditional and distinctive company vernacular was giving way to terms that formerly were used only in commercial companies.

Management structure became more formalized. In August 1968 the board named the company's first group of vice presidents:

R. P. Bourland, Administration
Doyle W. Ferguson, M.D., Medical Director
W. F. Hachmeister, Comptroller
Fred R. Higginbotham, Public Relations
Philip R. Overton, General Counsel
Charles D. Scott, Life Division
Rex L. Tidwell, Southern Region
Harley B. West, Marketing

Managers at all levels—supervisors, managers and executives—participated in a series of discussion sessions on principles of modern management designed by the American Management Association.

In December 1968 company staff salaries were put on the Hay system to more equitably determine salary levels. In 1969 the Training and Development Department was created. Job descriptions were prepared for each employee and evaluation committees reviewed all positions. Job grades were established, and salary ranges were assigned to make sure salary levels were competitive and equitable.

In the financial arena, agreements were reached with a local bank to transfer most of the company's investments so that they could be managed more assertively for profitability. An internal audit section was formed as well as a cost accounting section.

In marketing, West retired on March 15, 1969, and was replaced, effective a week later, by Victor R. Kennedy. "Vic" Kennedy joined the company in 1960 as a sales representative and worked his way up the ladder, becoming West's assistant enrollment director in 1968. Kennedy began to make his mark on sales, implementing sales performance standards, expanding sales training and enhancing marketing services to give the field force more support.

Technology moved ahead. In 1968 the company computerized membership and case history information. Up to that time, members' application cards were stored in the basement. The simple card listed the subscriber's name and number, group number, names of dependents and coverage. On the back of the membership card was the case card where incurred claims were listed by hand. Cards were retrieved frequently to verify someone's membership or coverage. Obviously, with hundreds of thousands of cards, the company was having difficulty keeping up with the information. Claims payment and answers to correspondence were sometimes delayed because an application card was misfiled. As a result of the new computerization, information was stored on a tape and was retrievable in hard copy.

In 1969 the company replaced the keypunch method of entering data into computers with new direct data entry technology that used cathode ray tube (CRT) terminals connected through communication lines to the mainframe computer. This increased the productivity about 30 percent. The company also opened an office known as Satellite No. 1 in leased space at LBJ Freeway and Midway Road that employed part-time workers (mainly retired typists and keypunch operators) to do the direct entry. The suburban location was a plus in attracting workers. Management began to plan for an automated claims processing system.

In 1970 the Michigan, Illinois, Florida and Texas Plans entered into a pooled information management arrangement known as MIFT. Each Plan undertook the development of a system module and coordinated its module with the other Plans. Illinois developed claims; Florida, finance; Michigan, payroll, personnel and production, planning and control; and Texas, membership. (The target date for completion of the system was 1973. The Texas Plan managed the Membership Administration Support System—MASS—which became operational in 1973, and the massive conversion of membership records began.)

Office space continued to be a challenge. The growth of staff and new business squeezed several departments out of the building. In March 1969 the board began considering construction of another building. They hired an architectural firm to survey various proposed sites and to proceed with appropriate economic and design studies. In addition to the downtown headquarters, the company leased space in the Hartford Building, Exchange Park, Dallas Federal and Taylor Street warehouse. By 1971 space in the Zale Building on Stemmons Freeway was also leased. Because of the fear of losing government contracts, the board decided in September 1971 to table the talk of the new building and continue leasing. By 1973 the downtown home office comprised less than half of the company's space around the city.

In 1971 a management consulting firm studied the company's organization structure and reported significant growth in the past five years: 28 percent increase in the number of people the company served, 140 percent increase in claims volume, 110 percent increase in the number of employees. The consulting firm reported that this growth demanded a more structured management staff.

The firm's plan recommended adding two new vice presidencies— Corporate Staff and Hospital Affairs. In January 1972 Kennedy was named to the former and Bill R. Newsom to the latter. Taking Kennedy's place as vice president of marketing was Wallace R. Langston, who had first joined the company as manager of the Case Department in 1949.

Kennedy's promotion put him on track toward becoming president. Beauchamp knew he would have to resign within the decade (in time for his sixty-fifth birthday in 1978), and he wanted to groom a possible successor. Kennedy was young, handsome, intelligent, to the point, and able to draw out the positive response of other people. He was, in a word, a leader. Beauchamp put Kennedy in charge of a corporate-wide reorganization of all areas. Throughout 1972 and 1973, Kennedy worked with company management in carefully honing organization structure, adding where it needed strength, clarifying goals and objectives, reducing staff when it was essential.

The workplace of the early 1970s saw several innovations. Employees were told in May 1971 that women could wear pantsuits, being defined as two or three pieces that were coordinated with tops extending to or slightly below the hipline.

Women were not only pioneering new ways of dressing professionally, they were advancing in the workforce beyond traditional roles. By 1972 a few more women in sales positions were gaining success: Jean Mauldin, Gail Norris and Rita Baker. In 1975 Lynda Melton was promoted to district sales manager of the Lufkin office, the first woman in sales management. The workforce was becoming more diverse racially as well as the company affirmed Equal Employment Opportunity in employment.

A larger workforce demanded more advanced communications. On May 14, 1973, the company switched to the Centrex phone system from the old operator switchboard. For the first time, every phone extension could be reached from the outside by direct dialing.

New products

Advances in product development helped the company maintain its marketing edge. On October 1, 1969, an out-of-hospital prescription drug program was implemented for the employees of the United Auto Workers, a national account. This program was a precursor to the later prescription coverage for regular business.

A new individual offering, the Texas Trail Blazer, went on the market on September 1, 1969. Those members of the old Comprehensive Service introduced in 1946 were allowed to transfer to Trail Blazer without meeting underwriting requirements.

During this period management began to talk about adding dental coverage to the list of products. Group dental coverage was offered in 1971 on a limited basis. In 1975 the company introduced the first major statewide coverage program: Denta-V, packaged in five components from basic to periodontics. It replaced the earlier dental contracts that were sold on a limited basis.

GLH had been slow in developing life insurance products but was now becoming a force in the life insurance industry. In a strategic effort to increase business, the company entered arrangements with other Plans in other states to sell companion life and disability benefits. In 1970 the company was licensed in Wyoming, Arkansas and Georgia. In 1973 New Mexico was added to the list and in 1976, Oklahoma. (In 1980 the company also marketed in Arizona and Nevada.)

Another major health product was introduced in 1976, Comprehensive Blue Cross and Blue Shield (CBC). Custom Coverage, because of its many choices for coverage levels, as well as many older coverages, had all become somewhat complicated to members. Supplemental coverages required a member to file under regular coverage and then perhaps major medical or accidental coverage. CBC wrapped its benefits into one program. Modifications to the claims payment system put into operation in September made processing more automated.

To market the new products, an advertising campaign premiered in 1976. "Does Your Company Think Enough of You to Provide the Best?" asked the ads in newspapers across the state and in television spots, national newsweeklies and trade publications.

At the March 1973 board meeting, Overton reported on a new bill presented to the Texas Legislature. The Texas Association of Public

Employees was attempting to set up its own statewide coverage system. Under the new bill, a committee would select one carrier and one contract. Up to that time, each state department purchased health coverage on its own. Most state agencies had been covered by Blue Cross and Blue Shield of Texas. For several years the company had been developing strategies to better serve the market and had opened an Austin office dedicated to state agencies on March 1, 1970.

In 1975 Senate Bill 18 was passed, which created the Texas Employee Uniform Group Insurance Benefit Act, giving state employees a uniform program of life, accident and health insurance. In early 1976 the state issued the request for proposal for the program, which would take effect September 1, 1976. It was to cover state employees except those in state universities, who would be included a year later. The company assembled a task force, prepared a bid and sent it to the state. In June 1976 it was announced that the company had won the bid for the uniform program. To manage the program, the company established the Austin Claims Service Center and a new claims processing section in Dallas. In a process of rebidding for the program in 1977, the company lost the business but regained it in 1980 and has had the group ever since.

Customer service enhanced

From the beginning, customer service was a priority with company departments, but this service was not centralized. As a result callers were frequently routed to several departments in an effort to get issues resolved. In 1973 the company made a major change by creating the Customer Service Center.

The center began operations in August 1973. It served as a point of contact for members (except for Medicare and Medicaid) who contacted the company through phone, letter or a visit. The center offered a one-stop, customer-oriented point of contact for members that provided access to all possible information on membership or claims. Jack Buzbee was the first manager of the area.

The Customer Service Center was made possible in part by the advent of new computer technology. For example, the membership system (the component that the Texas Plan managed in the MIFT consortium) made it possible to have instant access to membership information on CRT screens. Because several months were required to get all customer contact functions transitioned to the new area, it was April 1974 before the center was fully operational.

It was a time of dizzying change. As Beauchamp quipped to the board in 1973: "The spirit that I read in the top echelons of our organization these days could well be expressed as a slogan, borrowing that famous line, 'The past is prologue.' A free translation of that is, 'You ain't seen nothin' yet!'"[2]

The incessant escalation of health care costs was especially pressing. While health care inflation had been a topic since the post World War II days, it was a particularly relevant topic in the late 1960s and early 1970s. Health care technology was expanding as never before. A plethora of expensive and technology-intensive procedures were introduced that drove up the cost of care well beyond inflation. Each medical innovation carried an expensive price tag. Thanks to Medicare and Medicaid, more of the population was now receiving health care services, necessitating the need for more hospital beds, more equipment and more staff.

In the decade from 1960 to 1970, health care costs in Texas had more than doubled. By 1970 the average cost of a day in a Member Hospital was $75, and the average cost per case was $467.

Cost pressures began to change the nature of the health coverage business. Beauchamp told the board, "People are beginning to say to us, 'So you have a pretty good operation when it comes to rating the risk, collecting the premium, investing the money, and paying the claim, but that is not enough. We expect you to satisfy us that the claim you pay is right—the services you are paying for were actually needed and they carry a reasonable price tag!'"[3]

As health care costs claimed more and more of the nation's attention, the government began to require Medicare and Medicaid carriers to engage in a number of cost-saving measures. The company started conducting hospital audits. Utilization Review entered the company vernacular to describe a program to determine the medical necessity of hospital and physician care for the Medicare program. Government programs also stipulated a new way of determining reimbursement for medical and surgical claims: Usual, Customary and Reasonable Charge (UCR). This used a statistical formula to determine a range of what most physicians charged for specific procedures. The company began encouraging day surgery, and the use of freestanding ambulatory facilities in lieu of expensive inpatient hospitalization when warranted.

Some initiatives were tied to state or federal legislation. In a television address on Sunday, August 15, 1971, President Richard Nixon announced the Economic Stabilization Program, which froze wages and prices. Health insurers were allowed only limited rate increases. The wage-price freeze went through several phases until the controls were dropped on May 1, 1974.

Professional Standards Review Organizations (PSROs) were created by amendment to the Social Security Act in 1972. PSROs monitored government health care programs by setting utilization standards and by checking for abuses. In 1974 federal law set up the concept of Health Systems Agencies (HSA) across the nation. An HSA assessed a community's health care needs to avoid duplication of services. Texas was divided into twelve HSAs, and several company employees across the state served on their local panels. That same year the state legislature set up a certificate of need program that required a new hospital to certify the need for a new or expanded facility.

As new cost containment programs geared up, new ways of actually delivering health care services began. Various alternatives to traditional medicine became known in the company as alternative delivery systems, and a new division with that name was later formed with Ray Pace managing it.

In March 1973 the company ventured into an experimental arrangement with the Laredo-Webb County Health Department to participate in the Laredo Migrant Health Project, a federally funded pilot study to insure, initially, one hundred migrant families for a period of twelve months. The pilot study was to ascertain the cost of providing health care to a migrant population and to develop statistics for future migrant health care projects. It was highly successful and renewed for many more years.

In 1974 the Texas Plan began negotiations with the Bexar County Medical Foundation and partnered to open the Alamo Health Care Plan. It was the largest such venture in Texas between a group of doctors and a health care insurer. The company underwrote benefits, and care was provided by about five hundred physicians in the Bexar County/San Antonio area.

These various measures and programs began to affect the delivery of health care. In 1973 Beauchamp recalled the birth of his son many years earlier: "When my son was born, the hospital had a ten-day OB package deal that I bought at the time of admission. I guess it was standard practice. A doctor would probably be run out of the state, today, if he let one uncomplicated OB case stay ten days."[4] It was a different world.

Traditional relationships change

This different world made for different relationships between health care professionals and insurers. "We have inexorably been moved into a somewhat different relationship with the providers of health service," Beauchamp said at the time. "Certainly we have not been placed in the posture of an adversary—and heaven forbid that such a situation ever come about! But we are now expected to monitor the institutional and professional services purchased with our subscribers' dollars in such a way that we can effectively serve as guarantor of the validity of the purchase. The services must be actually delivered, of value proportionate to the price paid for them, and needed."[5]

The wedge between hospitals and Plans was beginning to be felt nationally as well. As Blue Cross Plans began to monitor hospital services more stringently in Texas, as across the nation, it became evident that the BCA would need to become independent from the AHA. In 1972 the two organizations finally agreed to separate, even transferring ownership of the Blue Cross name, service mark and standards of approval to the BCA.

The AHA insignia was removed from the center of the blue Geneva cross and replaced with a stylized human figure modeled on the well-known rendering of Leonardo da Vinci's universal man. The new symbol was introduced February 27, 1973. In April 1974 the new service mark replaced the old on the giant rotating sign on top of the downtown building.

The removal of the venerable AHA insignia became a manifest symbol that Blue Cross had matured. Birthed by hospitals, the movement was ready to leave home. Although at the grass roots level the working relationship continued successfully, Blue Cross had put the consumer in the center. (In 1979 the Texas Plan developed a new Member Hospital contract that eliminated the provision that hospitals guarantee the financial solvency of Blue Cross of Texas, completely relieving Texas hospitals of financial responsibility for the company.)

In 1978 the other service mark—the Blue Shield—got a facelift. To make the symbol discernible in smaller reproduction sizes, the snake lost its scales and the staff lost its wood grain. Together with the new Blue Cross symbol, the new service marks presented a more contemporary appearance.

In 1973 it was reported that the National Association of Blue Shield Plans was to be renamed the Blue Shield Association (BSA). By 1975 the executive committees of the BSA and BCA were meeting together regularly to better coordinate activities. Both associations realized that they needed to consolidate. Beauchamp himself authored the original resolution calling for consolidation of the two groups. The staffs of the two associations were consolidated on October 17, 1977, creating the Blue Cross and Blue Shield Association. (The new organization continued to have both a Blue Cross board and a Blue Shield board, however, until June 1982 when the boards were merged.)

Of all the changes of the time, none was more potentially radical than the change that national health insurance might bring upon the industry. The socialization of health care had been discussed ever since the beginning of the company in 1939, but in the 1970s it appeared that it was finally to be reality. Beauchamp predicted in 1972, "It is no longer open to speculation whether this country will have national health insurance. It will come, and the bets are that it will be next year. Even the form that it will take is beginning to crystallize." But this time around, the company was making some accommodations to the idea of socialized medicine. Beauchamp added, "There will be a role for us in this—a big role. We have to be gearing for it from here on in."[6]

Many were reporting that reliable estimates were now focusing on July 1, 1976, for the beginning of the plan. There were many varied proposals on how the program would be designed. "What will the nature of the program be?" mused Beauchamp.

> Total socialization, ala Kennedy? Catastrophic per the Long-Ribicoff design? Mandated for employees and free for the poor, as proposed by the (Nixon) Administration? Any of the several other schemes that are in the hopper? Whichever, the impact of Blue Cross and Blue Shield will be tremendous; if it is a government takeover we will be virtually out of business; if it creates a new market in a competitive environment we could be confronted with the necessity of vastly increasing our manpower and facilities. We are the best in the field, and we will rise to whatever requirements appear.[7]

As the decade progressed, however, the idea of a national health insurance program faltered. Financing methods couldn't be agreed upon, and President Gerald Ford (and Jimmy Carter after him) never really pushed assertively for it. It was eventually done in by the Reagan revolution of the early 1980s and the shift (in philosophy if not in actual practice) to private sector programs instead of government-regulated programs.

Growth in the mid-1970s

Company staff continued to grow, and new functions were added. Training and human resources activities grew to match the need, offering new training courses: supervisory management, correspondence training, claims examiner training, anatomy and coding training and data processing training, among others.

As changes continued in the health care sector, the company continued to hone its organizational structure and staff. In March 1973 Kennedy was named executive vice president, explicitly making him the apparent successor to Beauchamp.

In March 1974 L. M. Kennedy, D.D.S., president-elect of the American Dental Association, was named to the board. Dental was becoming an important new product line. In September of that year, Edward H. Carriker, D.D.S., who had been working as a dental consultant for the company, was named vice president/dental.

In the mid-1970s the Dallas labor market was tight, and the company had difficulty employing an adequate clerical staff. The decision was made to create an operation away from Dallas where the labor market was more promising, but it would have to be a self-contained function. In March 1974 a satellite installation in Denison was activated to code and enter Medicare Part B claims.

A second satellite operation opened in Bonham in December 1974. These two facilities, only twenty-six miles apart, each employed 127 people. Both were responsible for initial coding of Medicare Part B claims.

Regular business claims also decentralized into a self-sufficient operation. On July 6, 1974, the company opened a new facility in a leased space—the former Cook Discount Store building at the corner of Spring Valley and Central Expressway in Richardson. All regular business claims processing, employing 844 people, was under one roof and on one floor.

Data processing was taking a more commanding role in company operations as claims for both regular and government business escalated. The company had been contracting with EDS for data processing because Medicare and Medicaid had overtaxed the company's capability. The contract provided for turnkey data processing of Medicaid and Medicare Part B and lease of machine time for company staff to run regular business and Medicare Part A claims. The company began to build its own data processing capability and assumed responsibility for its own systems on November 1, 1975. The company purchased computers that were installed in space leased at the EDS operations building on Forest Lane. The separation was successful and on schedule.

The biggest change in company staffing structure occurred in July 1975 when senior vice presidents were added to the growing company organization chart. A new level of executive staff was needed to better administer the increasingly large and complex operations of the company. The board appointed Aune, Hachmeister and Langston as senior vice presidents. This was a continued effort on Beauchamp's part to have fewer staff reporting to him and to encourage decision making and leadership at other levels.

In February 1976 the company was stunned with the news that Vic Kennedy had died. His rise to leadership had been meteoric and his death just as sudden. About a year and a half earlier, he had been diagnosed with lymphoma and was under treatment. He had been on a track toward the presidency of the company, and his death left a significant hole in executive staff. Adding to the shock of his passing was that he was a widely respected and friendly man who exhibited rare leadership qualities. (One of Kennedy's children, Dan, who was eleven when his father passed away, eventually carried forth the Kennedy legacy, joining the company in 1990 as a sales representative assigned to Austin.)

In March several officers were summoned to the executive dining room on the twelfth floor of the downtown building. Hachmeister was one of the men and was surprised to learn when he arrived at the meeting that he had been named executive vice president. Hachmeister and Beauchamp had a good working relationship, but it was sometimes marked by disagreements, and the choice surprised many people.

At the same board meeting, Bill R. Newsom was named senior vice president to succeed Hachmeister.

In May 1976 Rogers K. Coleman, M.D., was hired as associate medical director, reporting to Louis Conradt, M.D. Coleman was a physician in Brownwood and also chief of staff at Brownwood Community Hospital. He joined the company for a respite from private practice, not really intending to stay with the company. One of his initial tasks was working on reasonable charge reimbursement in the Medicare program.

Strategic communications

Throughout the mid-1970s the public's concern about health care costs and the costs of government-sponsored health care programs resulted in the company (as was true of other Blue Cross and Blue Shield Plans) being in the public spotlight more frequently. Beauchamp wanted the company to do a better job of telling its own story and in 1975 he hired Jim Crawford, vice president and corporate secretary of the Dallas Chamber of Commerce, to develop the Corporate Communications Division.

Crawford pulled together several company functions into one strategic division that could better respond to the communication needs of a new era. In June 1976 it became operational. Elaine Vandygriff (later Gwaltney) was hired from the Training Department as the new director of public information. Longtime company artist Bob Kimbrell, manager of Merchandising (later named Graphic Productions), was moved under Crawford's management. Brents Broyles had been handling advertising, and he, too, moved to the new division.

The new division began an assertive communication program to employees and also developed better ways of responding to inquiries from the press. In addition, the division was especially helpful in adding communications polish to several task forces that had been meeting to develop proposals for important large pieces of business such as the state employees' group.

One of the first jobs of the new division was to announce to the public that the company had lost the Medicaid contract. The contract was being re-bid and the company had issued a proposal in April to the State Welfare Department. One of the competing bidders was EDS. The state at first suggested that the two companies file a joint bid, since each had expertise in different areas, but negotiations later broke down and the contract was not awarded to the Texas Plan. The contract expired on December 31, 1976.

It was the first time the company had lost a significant government contract. It was to be followed, a year later, with another loss, that of the state employees group (which the company recaptured in 1980). Gene Aune was the executive who had negotiated with the welfare department through the days of the former Old Age Assistance program to the Medicaid program. Aune recalled that losing Medicaid as well as the state group a year later were watershed events in the company's psyche: "That was a major blow to us. We had done a good job, plus we had a couple of hundred people involved in that. Until that time we had suffered no major defeats or losses."[8]

Several significant retirements occurred during this era. In September 1976 Boone Powell retired from the board. In March 1977 Phil Overton announced his wish to retire at the end of the year. At the time he was the only employee left who had been with the company from the very start, even before it was a company. Overton's contributions to the company were legion. He was most remembered for being the one who drafted the initial legislation—the enabling act—which allowed the company to form.

In September 1977 Wally Langston retired. Fred Rodgers was named to take his place as senior vice president. Veteran board member Tol Terrell also announced his retirement. In April 1978 board chairman James Aston asked to be relieved of his duties, and Fort Worth boot magnate John S. Justin, Jr. was named chairman of the board. To solidify Hachmeister's track toward the company's top staff office, the board named him president-elect. Beauchamp had firm plans to retire at the end of 1978.

Landmark status

Another company veteran was honored in 1978, but this time the honoree was not a person. The familiar rotating sign atop the downtown building was granted landmark status by the Dallas City Council in August 1978—but not without controversy.

In 1973 a city ordinance passed that prohibited rooftop signs in the central business district. Signs had to be removed by 1983 unless a sign had historical landmark status. In 1978 the City Plan Commission denied the sign's landmark status, but on appeal to the Dallas City Council, the company was awarded special status for the sign. It was argued that one reason the sign (and even the building) enjoyed this status was that former Dallas Mayor Bob Thornton had urged Beauchamp when he was on the city council to incorporate a "giant landmark sign" into the construction of the building. At the time Beauchamp recalled, "We never had a city council meeting that Mayor R. L. Thornton didn't ask me how we were coming on the building. He was gung-ho about that sign. He saw it as a civic ornament; a symbol of progress."[9] Also, it was explained to the city council that Beauchamp worked with the Central Business District Association to encourage building owners to remove unslightly overhanging signs. He practiced what he preached, for the company had removed the flashing message sign from the north side of the building.

The sign with the rotating service marks was the fourth in Dallas to receive historical status. It joined the flying red Pegasus atop the former Magnolia building, the clock on the Mercantile Bank building and the spire of the Republic Bank building.

D Magazine, however, couldn't resist a final jab at the company sign. One issue gave the city council a "thumbs down" for the declaration. "If a sign as ugly as that can be protected, why have an ordinance? Next thing you know, the council will be landmarking the Golden Arches."

As the famous Blue Cross and Blue Shield of Texas sign was getting historical landmark status, the company was looking to the northern suburbs to expand operations. In July 1976 the company purchased eleven acres and the 107,000 square-foot existing building at the corner of Spring Valley and Central Expressway in Richardson. The building was one of several satellite claims processing facilities. Adjacent to that property were twenty-nine additional acres available for purchase. For some time company leadership debated the pros and cons of centralization and decentralization, given the downtown building's lack of space.

In June 1978 the board voted to expand the Richardson facility, while maintaining the downtown building as corporate headquarters. The board approved the design and constructionof a new three-story structure that would be connected to the existing one. Ground was broken for the new building on July 24, 1978. Beauchamp was not content to merely shovel a few clumps of earth symbolically. He actually scooped the first piece of earth with a bulldozer after having had a brief lesson on how to operate the big machine.

It was one of his final public appearances as president of the Texas Plan. Beauchamp retired on December 31, 1978, after almost thirty-five years, ten of which were as president. A gala dinner was held on November 8. In honor of Beauchamp's retirement, the board of directors of both the BCA and BSA changed their meeting from Chicago to Dallas. At the head table that evening were dignitaries from across the System, including presidents from six Plans and even BCBSA President Walter

McNerney.

The Beauchamp years were years of growth for the company and filled with dramatic changes. With his level-headed and methodical approach to leadership, Beauchamp guided the corporation through a decade of exceptional challenges and innovations. He left the company with what he considered one of his most important legacies—a dramatic increase in the company's reserves.

As Beauchamp had steered the company into a more modern era with numerous progressive changes to the corporation, so Hachmeister would initiate many changes that he hoped would bring the company more fully into the contemporary health care marketplace.

Unfortunately, no one at the time could predict the challenges just ahead—challenges that would almost shut down the historic health care giant.

11 | 1979-1981: Taking Risks

"We have to maintain flexibility as the organization changes or as the demands of the marketplace change. We have to change. We can't continue to be what we were."
Walter F. Hachmeister

Walter F. Hachmeister assumed office as president on January 1, 1979. His first week was, in his words, "cursed with bad weather." However, inside the company all signs pointed to a vigorous and healthy year. In fact, the company was beginning what would be a banner year in its history. "Give Your Company the Benefit of the Best" heralded the new advertising theme. Indeed, Blue Cross and Blue Shield of Texas was perceived both inside and outside the company as the best in the industry.

Hachmeister began his tenure following more than twenty years with the Blue Cross and Blue Shield System. He was born August 30, 1920, in Chicago and graduated from Northwestern University with a bachelor's degree in accounting. During World War II he was a captain in the Army Air Corps. Before joining the Blue Cross Commission in 1957, he worked in finance with several firms. In 1961 McBee hired him as assistant comptroller. He moved up the management ranks, becoming comptroller in 1965, vice president/comptroller in 1968, vice president/finance in 1969, senior vice president in 1975 and was named executive vice president in 1976 and president elect in 1978.

He was profiled in the January 1979 issue of the employee magazine *Advance* and there he set the tone for his leadership. "I have also explained to Mr. Beauchamp," he told the magazine interviewer, "that while I will do my best to fulfill any commitments he has made, I do not feel honor bound to do so. If I feel that a direction should be changed or a policy should be adjusted or amended, I will do my best to do it."[1]

He was a president who was willing to take risks. In his first address to the board, he framed his hopes for the organization in terms of the new building in Richardson:

> My activities during the first three months in the President's office have paralleled our building program in many ways. Similar terms apply to both. For example, "fast-tracking" certainly is an appropriate term, not only as a construction method but for the swift-paced, significant changes in the first quarter of 1979. Many projects have been occurring simultaneously, moving from the firm foundation of Mr. Beauchamp's presidency.
>
> Another descriptive term is "flexibility." We've incorporated flexibility of design into the new building, and we've moved flexibly with the winds of change by capitalizing on the company's sound financial position and secure foundation.
>
> Many of the changes are the result of "schematic designs," blueprints with less than detailed drawings, but always with a final result in mind. The designs are concepts from which architects and management can build a finished product, which in our case is a strong, healthier, more productive, more competitive company.
>
> Fast-tracking, schematic designs, flexibility—These are appropriate descriptive words for the first quarter of this year.[2]

Fast-tracking change

Hachmeister inherited a company that was stable and built on a firm foundation, yet he felt the company had to move ahead quickly to catch up with a vastly changing marketplace. He was convinced the company needed to hone its operations so that it would be more flexible and meet the challenges of the marketplace.

In the employee magazine in early 1980, he told employees: "We have to maintain flexibility as the organization changes or as the demands of the marketplace change. We have to change. We can't continue to be what we were."[3]

Unlike Beauchamp, who had a large executive staff that met every Monday morning, Hachmeister wanted a small, workable group of upper management. He felt that the numerous vice presidents and associated staff had made Beauchamp's staff meetings unmanageable. In an effort to make the organization "slim and efficient," he reorganized the top executive level to consist of himself and five senior officers to comprise the management council. The seniors included Gene Aune, Jim Wilson, Ed Pascasio, Fred Rodgers and Bill Newsom. Newsom resigned in April, reducing the management council to four senior vice presidents.

Hachmeister realized that the biggest need was for a better information system. "The one area where we were terribly deficient was in data processing. We were handicapped by budget constraints—we had old systems in place that had been patched and repatched and revised and we just needed to do something," he later recalled.[4]

It became clear that the way to get the system the company needed was to subcontract out for it. On February 26, 1979, Hachmeister, Ross Perot and other officers of both the company and EDS gathered to sign a contract for a completely automated claims processing system. Under the terms of the contract, Electronic Data Systems Federal (EDSF), a subsidiary of EDS, would assume all data processing for regular business (which excluded Medicare) effective March 1. EDSF would also acquire the company's data processing systems, equipment and about 300 employees. About 170 employees remained within the Texas Plan to handle Medicare processing.

Converting to the new system offered many advantages. The company could get the benefit of more advanced systems and improve the accuracy and timeliness of claims processing while eliminating the risk of maintaining and buying equipment that was constantly being refined. Also, the contract would avoid the problems of recruiting qualified staff and would fix costs at the current level.

Looking toward Richardson

Next to the data processing contract, the biggest company news was the new building in Richardson. Ground had been broken and construction started.

At first the company intended for the building to be an expansion of the Richardson data processing operations with headquarters maintained downtown. However, in early 1979 the board's executive committee began to realize that moving all employees to the Richardson site would be advantageous. Though it would mean losing the Blue Cross and Blue Shield presence downtown in a building that had become an architectural landmark (and the sign an actual historical landmark), the suburban location would give the company the advantages of improved recruiting and operations efficiencies.

In May the board called a special meeting to determine what to do. As a result of the EDSF contract and the transfer of about three hundred

employees to the subcontractor, additional space in the Richardson building was now available. Management was predicting a slowdown in the
rate of employee growth, also as a result of the EDSF contract, further
lowering space requirements.

Architect E. G. Hamilton of the Omniplan design firm had devised a
plan to add 92,000 square feet of finished space to the 432,000 square
feet previously approved. At first, the building was to be four stories with
the fourth floor's interior unfinished until future expansion plans called
for the additional space. The revised plan included finishing the fourth
floor, adding a second and partial third floor to the east wing, adding a
partial third floor to the west wing and increasing parking space in the
garage. The projected cost was $28.8 million. The board unanimously
approved the project.

Construction proceeded. At 5 p.m. on June 23, 1979, the construction crew was digging around the foundation of the existing building when
a steel beam supporting the existing building's slab gave way, causing
the slab to shift. Then, seventy-five feet of wall on the west end col-
lapsed, causing the data processing equipment to shut down. Luckily, no
staff members were injured (the accident occurred just thirty minutes
after most staff left for the day), but the computer hardware was left exposed to the elements.

About two hundred staff members from the company, EDSF, IBM, the
construction company and an electric company arrived on the scene to
begin restoration of the systems. The structure was covered in heavy
plastic sheeting where the masonry had fallen, allowing the crisis team to
begin recovery.

They worked throughout the night. To sustain the hardworking staff,
food was ordered from a small hamburger establishment across Central
Expressway. "We called them and said we needed 200 hamburgers and
cold drinks," Public Information Director Elaine Gwaltney recalled. "It
was the largest order they ever had!"[5] Staff was fed, worked through the
night, and by about noon the next day the system was back up and working, with the hole in the wall temporarily patched.

The design emerges

The building employed the "fast-track" design, which meant that
construction started before the design was completed. For example, even
though the architect had not finished designing the partitioning or se-
lecting the carpet, crews could start digging the basement and erecting
the precast concrete.

The prefabricated design made fast-tracking possible. The building
was designed with huge precast concrete "bents" as the integral struc-

ture. Bents were prefabricated steel-reinforced concrete beams that were U-shaped (or bent) and weighing 120,000 pounds each. They were connected together to create the massive concrete skeleton of the building. Bents were also an important design element on the exterior of the building. The first bent was placed on June 25, 1979, just two days after the wall fell on the existing structure.

While the downtown building was a monument (perhaps to a man— McBee—and at least to a movement), the Richardson building reflected the business realities of the day. In contrast to the downtown building, which was squeezed into a lot and thrust upward for twelve stories, the suburban building was long, lean and horizontal, more than double the size of the downtown headquarters. In fact it was as long as approximately one and one-half football fields.

The downtown building relied on heavy exterior ornament, while the Richardson building used its internal structure as its external face: spare, strong and honest. The concrete bents were left exposed. Long walls of glass attached to the bents created an interior workplace graced with natural light and yet protected from the elements with double-paned windows insulated with a vacuum pocket.

The core of the building that housed the escalators was crowned with large skylights, flooding the center of the building with natural light. Employees welcomed the escalators because they could move quickly across the expanse of the building instead of waiting on elevators that laboriously lugged downtown staff up and down twelve floors all day.

Inside, the offices were almost completely modular, with contemporary partition walls easily erected to accommodate a changing work force. Soft neutral colors were used: gray, ivory, tan and terracotta, accented by rich blue fabric on chairs as a contrasting highlight color. Fabric-covered partition walls absorbed sound so that employees could enjoy the advantages of an open system, but with privacy. New modern furniture was also purchased to be phased in over a two-year period.

The building was spare but beautiful in its simplicity and integrated in its construction. Recognition of the design came in April 1983 when it received a Merit Award from the Dallas Chapter of the American Institute of Architects.

While the building was being constructed, the sale of the downtown building didn't go as smoothly as first expected. In August 1979 it was announced that the building had sold, but the buyer backed out. (Finally, in October 1981 the building sold to a real estate development firm. The firm then stripped the building of its late 1950s-modern facade down to the steel skeleton and reskinned the building with a dark mirrored façade. The offices were then leased. It was a task akin to turning a frog into a prince, opined one local newspaper.)

All employees (with the exception of Medicare employees) were to be housed in the new Richardson building. The lease on the Zale Building was expiring, and Medicare employees moved to One Brookriver Center in the Stemmons Freeway area in late 1980.

Challenges of change

While the new building was being constructed during 1979, the company began to get a taste of the changing marketplace.

The Pregnancy Disability and Age Discrimination in Employment Act had been signed into law in October 1978 by President Jimmy Carter. It required that employers treat pregnancy and related conditions just as any other health condition for purposes of employment and benefits. The law was far-reaching for the company. Gone were flat rate maternity allowances under group health coverages, a nine-month maternity waiting period and specific exclusions for maternity benefits. Changing all group contracts to meet the provisions of the law was demanding. Likewise, the Age Discrimination Act was amended allowing workers to stay on the job to age seventy, which affected the company's groups, since most coverage either reduced or ceased at age sixty-five. Revising policy forms, endorsements and billings, as well as communicating the change to groups, was a major task throughout 1979. The first issue of *Group News*, a new quarterly newsletter to enrolled groups, was produced in an effort to communicate the changes.

Marketing operations realigned to become more aggressive. The Mid-Cities District Office was established to serve the growing areas between Dallas and Fort Worth, and regional territories were realigned and consolidated. In the home office, the underwriting function was placed under marketing to ensure more responsiveness to consumer demand in rate setting. Public attitude studies were commissioned, including one aimed at the group benefits buyer. A more aggressive marketing program of individual health and life products was begun. A new health product for small groups, The Ten-Plus Plan, was introduced, offering coverage up to one million dollars for groups that formerly could not purchase group coverage. Dental coverage continued to be a big seller. A Sales Promotion Department was also created.

As in the previous decade, the rising cost of health care remained the largest challenge of all, necessitating that cost containment remain a priority. The company had been active for several years in many elements of cost containment, such as nonduplication and coordination of benefits, hospital price negotiations, subrogation and workers' compensation, and fraud investigations.

Other cost containment activities included involvement in health planning, innovations in new benefits for pre-admission testing and free-standing surgical centers, and a strengthening of utilization review activity. A pilot phase of the pre-admission testing program was implemented in February 1979 at thirteen Member Hospitals. This was a voluntary agreement between the company and a Member Hospital in which diagnostic tests for an elective inpatient admission were performed on an outpatient basis in hopes of reducing the number of inpatient days with the associated costs.

The Texas Conference on Health Care was sponsored by the company and held in Dallas October 1-2, 1979, to explore issues of cost and access to health care under the theme of "Health Care Costs are Everybody's Business." The conference attracted several notable political and health care leaders of the day, including nationally known columnist and conservative intellectual William F. Buckley, Jr. Other speakers were Walter McNerney, president of BCBSA, the president of the AHA and the executive vice president of TMA.

That health care costs were, indeed, everyone's business was the thrust of a program called the Voluntary Effort, which was an attempt by the company in cooperation with Texas hospitals to reduce the increased rate of hospital costs.

Amid realigning itself for a changing marketplace, the company took time to acknowledge its heritage and commemorate Dallas as the birthplace of the national Blue Cross idea. In April the fiftieth anniversary of the Blue Cross concept kicked off in Chicago at the Blue Cross and Blue Shield President's Forum.

With the theme "Commemorating Fifty Years of Working for a Healthier America," the Texas Plan as well as Plans throughout the System commemorated a half-century of leadership in health care. Special presentations were made to Baylor Hospital and the Dallas Independent School District recognizing them for their part in the beginning of the concept.

Advances in the workplace

Several important and popular workplace programs were instituted in late 1978 and 1979:

- Flextime, introduced in 1978, was successful and popular among employees.
- Job posting was implemented in October 1978 to provide employees with more opportunity for promotion.
- In that same month, a comprehensive review of the corporate salary program was done, and salary ranges were subsequently adjusted

to become more competitive with salaries in business generally.

   •   The van pool program, recognized as a company necessity following the oil embargo that threatened to cripple national oil and gas supplies, started in 1979.

   •   The energy crisis even affected the company dress code. In order to set the thermostat at seventy-eight degrees during the summer, the company temporarily relaxed employee dress codes to permit exclusion of coat and tie for male employees when they were not in contact with the public.

In September the board approved the creation of political action committees (PAC) to involve employees more in the political process. Because of the complexities of creating a federal PAC, the board later decided to form a state PAC instead.

As 1979 drew to a close, it was apparent that the company had just completed one of the best years of its history.

The year was extraordinary for marketing. The company had sold more than twice the number of health and dental groups than in any previous year. Individual and life products also showed significant advances. Financially it was also a banner year—the most successful in history. Comptroller Vernon Walker told a pleased board that at the end of the year the company had achieved net income of $25.5 million for the year (which was $19.5 million more than at the end of 1978).

The building was progressing, and it was hoped that the move could occur at the end of 1980. Employee benefits were enhanced with dental added to the basic health package and the retirement plan improved. Among enrolled groups, health care utilization figures showed a slight dip. As company employees celebrated the new year of 1980, all indications were that everything was looking better than ever at the Texas Plan.

Converting to the new system

The staffs of both the company and EDSF began to prepare for the massive conversion months in advance. Employees learned the new programming language and the theory associated with the new system. Benefits had to be "strung"—coded into the system so that it could know how to pay benefits according to various contracts. To handle these new tasks, the company created the Benefit Coding Department. The fledgling department had to analyze some twenty thousand contracts to code the system properly. The department also had to track down all the memos, notations and exceptions for all contracts to be sure benefits could be paid as promised.

On September 4, 1979, the company implemented the first phase of the system—the entry format change that gave entry operators a chance to familiarize themselves with the requirements of the new system. This resulted in a backlog of claims, which was quickly reduced. At various times between February 8 and February 19, 1980, eight different claims payment systems were turned off. To be ready for the startup of the final phase in March, claims had to be cleared out of the old system. New claims received from mid-February to March 3 were entered into the new claims system and held until the system was on.

The beginning of the year was normally heavy for members to file their own claims. The company sent a postcard to members who submitted their claims during this period, explaining that their claims would be processed as soon as the new system was converted.

On March 3, 1980, conversion to the new regular business claims processing system entered its final phase as the system was activated. The old patchwork of claims payment systems was now completely off.

But within weeks it was apparent something was wrong. The new system was extra-sensitive to check charges to ensure proper benefits and payments for each claim. It was soon apparent that the sensitivity of the system was causing about one-third of the claims to fail the edits and so large numbers of claims were suspended for manual review and re-entry.

By April Fred Rodgers told the board that they had underestimated the complexity of the system, the effect of conversion during the winter peak season for claims and the extensive training effort required. As the backlog of claims increased, Hachmeister temporarily realigned some of the responsibilities of senior staff to better manage the conversion. Aune was temporarily given claims so that Rodgers could concentrate on conversion.

Not only was the system slow in paying claims but it was also making mistakes in claims payments, causing a high degree of frustration among members. The number of calls to the Customer Service Department was increasing at a phenomenal rate. By June the department was handling three thousand calls daily. Additional personnel were pulled from other areas to help handle the calls. Dallas media began to take notice, and a front-page story in June in the *Dallas Morning News* pointed out that customers were having a hard time getting through.

At the executive committee meeting of June 27, Aune reported on the situation. "I don't know whether to give an optimistic report, pessimistic report, or somewhere in-between," he told the committee.

"Give it to us honestly, Gene. We want the straight dope," responded one officer.

Aune proceeded to do just that. He described the backlog of about two and one-half weeks worth of claims in a state of suspense. "New fresh claims are going through very effectively," he told the committee, "but unfortunately there is still residue that we are battling there—claims for some reason or other did not make the conversion from the old system into the new system, claims that keep recycling and have to be pulled out and handled individually."

Marketing senior vice president Wilson expressed concerns about the effect the backlog was having on marketing efforts. "We have a lot of groups I consider in jeopardy position," he reported.[6] Indeed, the effects of the backlog began to show on cancellation reports. In June Wilson told the management council that the company had lost up to 15,000 contracts since the first of the year, and he thought it possible that yet another 180,000 might be lost if the claims problems weren't resolved.

Operation cleanup

A concerted effort was aimed at clearing the backlog and correcting the system and thus reducing the customer service problems. Employees and management hunkered down for the task. It was a mammoth job, since every day the division received more than twenty thousand claims.

The Suspense Department reorganized to handle claims that were kicked out of the system for manual review. In May 1980 it had a log of about 250,000 items of suspense. Within sixty days, employees had lowered that to 45,000, only two and one-half days of receipts. Several new departments were created to better manage the process—Quality Control, Dental, Special Groups, Adjustments.

A new phone system was installed in August that would further decrease the customer service problems by improving access for the increased number of calls. Phone lines were increased from 60 to 200. A leased facility on Royal Lane and Central Expressway was opened to house 240 employees in the Customer Service and Individual departments.

Employees clocked in many hours of overtime on nights and weekends. Vacations were shortened, postponed or even canceled.

Through the spring months of 1980, average claims turnaround time was more than two weeks. In June average processing time was more than three weeks, but by August it was down to ten or eleven days, and by October a mere seven days. Customer service calls also decreased, following the claims processing improvement.

Despite the advances, claims backlogs remained a problem, and the system, though improving, still was not functioning as hoped. Groups were continuing to leave because of service problems. Financially, the outlook was bleak. By July the books were showing a twelve million dollar loss.

Despite the problems surrounding the system conversion in 1980, the company made progress in other areas during the year.

Sales throughout the year actually did well. New sales were healthy despite heavy cancellations. By the end of the first six months, thirty-seven thousand more contracts than the previous year were sold.

The biggest sales boost of the year came in June with the announcement that the company had recaptured the State of Texas employees account. The program covered more than 100,000 employees and retirees and was to begin September 1. Part of the contract with the state was to set up an Austin office dedicated to the group, which Bob English would head up.

In April the company purchased a private airplane. The executive committee agreed that a state the size of Texas could justify the purchase.

In January the company had issued a request for proposal for data processing for Medicare Parts A and B, to begin in April 1981. In September it was announced that EDSF was the successful bidder for that system as well.

Besides converting to a new data processing system, technology was advancing in other areas. The Provider Automation Department began, which allowed tape-to-tape claims filing, avoiding much of the paperwork problems. Three hospitals had the program in March 1979, and by February 1981 computer terminals were installed in seventy-one hospitals with thirty-six on the waiting list. Physician offices were also beginning to understand the advantage of filing claims electronically. A pilot program with doctors ended in July 1980 and was deemed successful enough to begin active marketing of the service to doctors.

As the year drew to a close, the new building was ready for its first occupants. Move-in occurred over a space of several months so as not to disrupt daily business. The first departments to move on December 22, 1980, were the Medical and Provider Affairs divisions. Moving vans traveled up and down Central Expressway for months until move-in of all departments was complete in early 1981.

Chaos

During the first quarter of 1981, statistics about the preceding year were gathered, and it became clear that the company was in trouble.

Despite the company's best efforts, a serious claims backlog still existed. The company took several measures to alleviate the situation. For example, one weekend employees throughout the company were invited to help audit claims and received a cash bonus for doing so. Cash flow was such a serious problem that Vernon Walker recalled sending staff to the bank every hour with premium checks received to cover claims payments being made. Customer service problems abounded with underpayments, overpayments and duplicate payments. Public confidence was eroding.

While the system conversion was the catalyst for the difficulties, several other factors entered into the picture. Health care utilization spiked dramatically in 1980 for all insurers, aggravating financial losses. The earlier decision to put underwriting under marketing boosted sales but damaged long-range finances because some groups had not been rated as high as necessary. Aggravating the financial picture was the fact that the new building was being financed with cash, a decision that was made during the financial windfall of 1979. By 1981 cash was severely limited.

Investments couldn't easily be turned into cash. Inflation went sky high, and the company's investment portfolio was hurt in the process. As inflation increased, the company's bonds were devalued and their liquidity suffered. Bonds were shown on the books at their face value. If they were sold, they had to be listed at the selling price—and at the time they were valued at about half of their face value. As a result the bonds were worth more on paper if they were not sold.

Hachmeister first told the board in February that the company lost $24.6 million in 1980, but soon it became apparent that the losses would be even greater. How great was not yet known.

Recognizing that drastic measures were necessary to save the company, the board became more involved. Media attention continued. Both Dallas newspapers carried frequent stories about the company, many of which were picked up on newswires and transmitted across the state. Comments reflecting the public's anxiety accompanied each news report. Groups continued to cancel in large numbers. Rumors were circulating that the company was close to insolvency and would perhaps be closed by the state insurance board.

One winter day in late 1980 or early 1981, Vernon Walker recalled sitting in his corner office on the third floor of the new building with one of his employees, Roy Kennedy. The two gazed out the windows overlooking the northeast section of the campus, landscaped with young trees that stood bare in the frigid season.

"How are we going to handle this?" Kennedy asked.

"I don't know," Walker responded. "Maybe it's time I start worrying about my next job."

"We might have some time," Kennedy sighed with perhaps a scant amount of hope.

"Yes, Roy, but I'll bet you money we'll never see the leaves hit those trees in the spring."[7]

Throughout the company at all levels, employees were beginning to understand that despite a long history of serving the state, there were no guarantees that the company could survive this trauma.

A regular board meeting was scheduled on March 28 and, as usual, the executive committee was to meet the day before. Board chairman John Justin called members of the executive committee and told them that he felt the company needed new leadership and that he wanted to call for Hachmeister's resignation. All agreed.

On March 27 Justin went to Hachmeister's office in the north building. (The president's office in the east wing was not yet finished.) Justin asked for his resignation. "Fine, you've got it," Hachmeister replied calmly and then drafted the letter of resignation.[8]

Hachmeister walked up to the executive committee meeting to present the letter. Aune recalled that the senior officers were asked to wait in an outside area before the meeting. Hachmeister went in and a few minutes later came back out. "Gene," he said, walking over to Aune, "the executive committee wants to see you." Aune stood to follow Hachmeister, assuming the two were going into the meeting together. But Hachmeister stopped at the doorway, ushered Aune into the room, and then closed the door. Aune faced the executive committee alone.

Justin asked him if he would be willing to be the acting president and CEO. One board member laughed, "Well, maybe Gene needs a cup of coffee to swallow that one!" perhaps using humor as a defense against the drama of the moment.

"I'll do whatever I can," Aune answered resolutely. I'll give it a go."[9]

Hachmeister arrived home and announced the news to his wife Mary Lee. "I just felt like the weight of the world had been lifted from my shoulders," he later remembered. Though the immediate pressure was gone, he began dealing with the frustration and disappointment of not being able to redirect the company in a time of change. "I just couldn't seem to get the organization in high gear where I thought it should be," he remembered.[10]

Now, it was another man's turn to get the organization in high gear.

Gene Aune was a thirty-two year veteran of the company. He had joined Blue Cross and Blue Shield of Texas in 1949 as a clerk in the Service Department, (underwriting and marketing) and began moving up the ranks. In 1970 he was named vice president of public relations (state and government relations) and then in 1975 senior vice president of government programs.

One of his early tasks was trying to restore public confidence. On May 28 he held a press conference to state that the company was solvent and would continue to pay claims. What perhaps helped hold public concern at bay the best was a news release Aune brought from the State

Board of Insurance that said the department was satisfied about the solvency of the company. Examiners were on site at headquarters to monitor operations, and the state insurance commissioner was now requesting regular reports to assure its solvency.

By April the auditors reported that the 1980 financial situation was worse than thought—the company had actually lost $47.3 million. An amended financial statement was filed with the state insurance department.

The executive leadership focused on monitoring the company's cash situation, managing the claims processing system and trying to recoup overpayments. Aune instructed management to analyze all staffing and budgets and reduce expenditures. Management consultants were hired to advise executives on developing a strategy to revive the company. The company changed outside auditors.

Throughout all this activity, Aune found the role of acting president difficult. The transitional nature of the job prevented him from making some of the decisions that had to be made. New leaders were needed, but he found it difficult to hire anyone, not knowing who would eventually become president.

The company had yet another systems conversion to face. The Medicare system, which had also been subcontracted out, began conversion on May 4. This conversion also resulted in a backlog of claims, but this time the company was more prepared, and inventory was eventually reduced to normal levels.

Public and media attention continued to be focused on the struggling company. In June the *Dallas Times Herald* titled a story with the puckish headline, "Singing the Blue Cross Blues," illustrated with a cartoonish Aune drowning in a blue sea with a storm brewing overhead.

Despite such heavy attention from the media, company leaders hunkered down to manage the claims situation and increase efforts to pursue collections of erroneous payments. An executive search firm was hired for an expeditious search for a president. The board's finance committee very carefully managed investments, making the best of the company's portfolios. In an effort to improve the severe cash shortage, the executive committee suggested hiring a realty company to pursue a sale/leaseback arrangement for the new building.

The calendar dragged along through the summer into the fall. About the first of October, Aune visited Justin in his Fort Worth office. Justin told him that they were going to hire a management consultant to try to make sense of the chaos. "We're going to bring in a fellow that really understands finance," Justin told Aune. "His name is John Melton."[11]

12 | 1981-1990: Turnaround and Transition

"I question my intelligence, but I am here, and
I sure expect to succeed."
John D. Melton

Throughout the chaotic months following the president's resignation, Justin stayed in contact with the State Board of Insurance, traveling to Austin once a week to keep the agency informed of company progress. The state board watched the company closely. In Justin's words, "They had that hatchet ready to drop and take over."

State Board Chairman Bill Daves told Justin about a man named John Melton. "If anybody can pull you out, he can," he told Justin. Melton would make a good consultant and troubleshooter, Daves suggested. Melton was retired, living somewhere in East Texas on a lake, but perhaps he could be convinced to come out of retirement.

So Justin called Melton. He introduced himself and invited him to lunch.

"No," Melton replied.

"Why?" Justin asked.

"I know who you are and what you want, and I know what your problems are and I don't want any involvement in it." Melton had already been contacted by the State Board of Insurance about the situation at the Texas Plan.

"Oh, I'm not that bad of a fellow," Justin said, trying to inject humor into the tenseness of the conversation. "I'll pay for lunch myself, and I'll try not to be too bad."

"I'm tired and I'm retired and I like what I'm doing, and I don't want to get involved in any type of business," Melton persisted.

"I understand that," Justin said, dropping the humor. "But I need help. I'm in a terrible jam at Blue Cross and Blue Shield of Texas. This is an important thing for the state of Texas, and I need all the help I can get. The least you can do is have lunch with me."

The conversation went back and forth. Melton was concerned that they would be seen in public and thus fuel rumors. Justin promised to get a private dining room. Melton relented and agreed to lunch on the next day.

Justin then called a club and requested a private dining room for the meeting, but on such short notice no room was available. There was, the receptionist said, a ballroom available. "How many are you expecting for lunch?" she asked. "Two," he replied, saying he would take the ballroom.

"You don't understand, sir. This is a huge room."

"I don't care. I have to have a private room."

So a ballroom was reserved for a cozy lunch for two.

The next day, Justin arrived at the club. "I went in and they had put a 10- by 12-foot beautiful rug in the middle of this ballroom and two beautiful chairs and a table and flags, the American and Texas." The table was set in the middle, not at an end, of the cavernous room. In a moment John Melton came in, strode across the expanse of the ballroom floor and began their meeting.

Justin remembered the conversation. "John and I talked and talked. He said, 'I'm retired, I don't want anything to do with it.' I told him, 'I'll help you any way I can.' Well, I was waving the American flag and singing the *Star Spangled Banner* and *Eyes of Texas* and offering apple pie. I bared my chest to him, that Blue Cross and Blue Shield of Texas is in trouble, that it was a fine organization and it's just a shame to let it go down the drain."

Justin recalled that the lunch was hot when it left the kitchen but definitely cooling by the time the waiter arrived at the table in the middle of the ballroom floor.

Justin persisted in his harangue.

Finally, Melton agreed to come on as a consultant. "But I don't want to work with anybody but you. I'll report to the board, but I'm going to depend on you to be my liaison with the board. If I come in there I'm going to do a lot of things in a hurry and I'm not going to be able to call the board every time I want to do something," Melton insisted.

Justin agreed to those terms and Melton was hired. Justin went home knowing he had done perhaps the biggest selling job of his long career. "If you sell cowboy boots," Justin recalled years later with the legendary twinkle in his eyes, "you've got to be a pretty good salesman." Anybody who could pull John Melton out of retirement for what seemed an impossible job was indeed a good salesman.[1]

The Melton era begins

At the board meeting on September 26, 1981, Justin announced that John D. Melton, retired president of Republic National Life Insurance Company, had been employed as a special management consultant effective October 1, 1981. It became evident that the company needed a permanent president as quickly as possible to hire qualified senior officers who could lead the company. On October 14 Justin met with Melton again and offered him the job of president. This time it didn't take a ballroom or even a dinner to convince him.

On October 19 a special meeting of the board was called. Justin told the board that the executive committee recommended Melton as president, effective immediately. The committee also suggested that Aune remain with the company as executive vice president. The board unanimously affirmed both men.

Melton came to the company with a firm record of achievement in leading insurance companies, but he fell into that track quite by accident. He was born December 1, 1925, in Winnfield, Louisiana. His first job was at age fifteen as a stick boy in a lumber yard in that community. "It was hard work," he recalled, "but I was making 25 cents an hour, so I figured I'd retire soon anyway." He arrived in Texas courtesy of the military and was stationed in Waco. There, he met his future wife, Norma, a student at Baylor University. Melton had two stints with the U. S. Air Force, from 1943 to 1945 and then from 1951 to 1953. Between those engagements he married Norma and came to Dallas to earn a bachelor's degree in accounting from Southern Methodist University. Once he was discharged from his duties in the Korean conflict, he began his insurance career.

He hadn't really planned on insurance as a career. "At the time I was discharged, I had a wife, a four-year-old son, and another child due to be born any day, and I needed a job. The first job that was offered to me was with an insurance company. That's just how much planning ahead I did on my insurance career."[2]

That first job was with Reserve Life Insurance Company. He left that company in 1969 as vice president of finance. He then was president of the Hawaii Corporation Insurance Group in Honolulu for three years and then returned to Texas in 1973 as a consultant for the State Board of

Insurance. The state board sent him as a consultant to Republic Life Insurance Company in Dallas and in 1977 he became president of that company. In 1981 he retired briefly to East Texas until John Justin romanced him back into the business.

Melton was a no-nonsense man. He was tough and he was fair. He had an ability, perhaps learned in his education and experience in finance, to see the bottom line of any argument quickly and get right to the point. He smoked incessantly and unapologetically.

The situation he entered as president of the troubled Texas Plan was reminiscent of the past. Like McBee, Melton came in to save a faltering organization on the brink of collapse. Like Beauchamp, he had experience with the State Board of Insurance and was an insurance insider. Like, perhaps, Justin Ford Kimball, he was direct and even gruff, though probably with a more developed sense of humor than Kimball.

Melton was not a visionary. He was basically a financial man with a keen sense of getting through the garbage of a situation gone awry and making it work again.

He was no-nonsense with reporters as well. In one of his first interviews following the announcement of him becoming president, he told the *Dallas Morning News*, "I'm satisfied the company is completely solvent, and that it can remain solvent. But it will take a hell of a lot of work." Elsewhere in the same story he said, "Camelot is over as far as Blue Cross is concerned. It was a great place, but it can no longer be afforded."[3] He later explained to employees that he was referring to earlier days when "the company was buying airplanes, building buildings and spending money very freely."[4]

The *Dallas Morning News* later described him as a man "known in Dallas insurance circles for his surgical skills on ailing companies," who entered the "inner sanctum of Blue Cross and Blue Shield of Texas in (the) fall and decided his chances of salvaging the problem-plagued company were pretty good."

The story quoted Melton, "I question my intelligence, but I am here, and I sure expect to succeed." The comment reflected his dry humor, honesty and prediction of the future of the company. "I want to see this company back to where it was—a real viable part of the health care industry in Texas."[5]

Melton's first office was hardly luxurious. It was a small room (it later became a stock closet) in the north building while workers put the finishing touches on the executive offices in the east wing. He often worked out a problem by pacing, but his office was too small to walk in, so he paced outside his office. Carolyn Colley, then corporate secretary, recalled that he was always pacing. "Every time I went over to the copy machine outside his office, there he was—pacing back and forth, deep in thought on how to turn the company around."[6]

The pacing continued and a plan developed.

He began by holding executive committee meetings monthly so that the leadership of the company could stay on top of the situation. He asked for and got permission to hire senior financial and marketing officers without prior approval of the executive committee. He suggested that the company plane be grounded. The executive committee had already decided to sell it and its hangar.

By November Melton had hired Ross Snyder as chief financial officer and Mickey Greene as chief marketing officer. They joined Ed Pascasio, Jack Ponder and Gene Aune as the senior executive team.

The most serious situation facing the new management team was the company's lack of cash and low surplus. If it wasn't improved immediately, the company could go under. The corporate bond portfolio remained badly devalued and couldn't be liquidated.

To buy some time, Melton convinced the State Board of Insurance to delay reviewing the company's financial statement for two months. Then, he had the land at the Richardson headquarters appraised. The appraisal showed that the value of the land had increased by eleven million dollars, which could be shown on the balance sheet as surplus.

Also helping the cash situation was a reinsurance agreement with Southwestern Life Insurance Company in Dallas, which purchased twenty million dollars of individual life from the books of GL&H. (It was later repurchased in two $10 million increments in 1985 and 1986.) The agreement with Southwestern Life was made on the last day of 1981, just in time to show the increased cash on the books.

The downtown building had sold on October 16 and that also relieved the cash situation somewhat. Melton began to look for a buyer for the Richardson building who would then lease back the property to the company.

While those actions helped the cash situation, the senior officers also were faced with the necessity of doing a better job of managing benefits payments. In November Melton went to the hospital relations committee of the board and asked for a 9.9 percent maximum increase in negotiated hospital charges for 1982. In December he appeared in front of the THA board to present his plan for the hospital cap, and all agreed that it was a wise course of action.

To rein in medical-surgical costs, Melton decided it was high time the company instituted the Usual, Customary, and Reasonable (UCR) method of paying for physician charges. Though UCR had been included as a provision in regular business contracts since the 1970s, it had not been implemented. Melton went to Austin again to present the UCR plan to the TMA. UCR went into effect on February 15, 1982, dubbed Reasonable Charge in the company's marketing literature.

Melton also led the effort to rein in internal costs. The company had been involved in CABCO (Combined A and B Consortium)—a multi-Plan effort to develop systems to process Medicare Parts A and B claims. The project was first conceived in 1977 and begun in 1978, but did not coalesce as quickly as hoped and had begun to be a financial drain on the Texas Plan. The company withdrew participation in CABCO in late 1981.

Melton went on the road around the state, talking with hospitals and physicians and enlisting their effort to cut costs and protect policyholders. Though he encountered a few bumps in that road across Texas, most health care providers cooperated.

As Christmas 1981 approached, Melton began what became an annual ritual by making rounds in the company, giving each employee a handshake and greeting for the holiday. In his first year of holiday visits, he actually traveled to each offsite office to greet and shake hands with virtually every employee. In later years he abridged his holiday greetings primarily to the home office and some claims offices around the state.

A hopeful new year

As the new year of 1982 dawned, the mood was tentative but expectant. Melton announced to the executive committee in January that thirty-one million dollars had been added to reserves because of the life insurance ceding and appraisal of the building. Some hospitals were balking at the price cap, but all came around eventually. The UCR method of physician reimbursement began on February 15 and showed immediate savings.

Melton scheduled a press conference on Friday, February 26 at the downtown Press Club to provide 1981 financial data. Both Dallas papers led their stories with a bad news/good news angle. The company lost $36.1 million in 1981, but that was considerably less than the $47.3 million loss of 1980. Melton's attitude with reporters at the press conference was his usual down-to-earth manner, and reporters responded to his honesty.

Simultaneously with the press conference, employees were given the press release. On the following Monday, employees also were given a news release from the State Board of Insurance, assuring the public of the company's solvency. Melton wrote an accompanying memo, assuring them that the company was beginning the road toward recovery. "I am absolutely confident that Blue Cross and Blue Shield of Texas will be in business at this time next year and with your wholehearted support, 1982 will be the beginning of a long and prosperous future for our company."[7]

Confidence was again beginning to show in the company. The cover of the April issue of the employee magazine *Advance* showed a sun rising over the headquarters alongside a rainbow, with storm clouds receding and the headline, "Here comes the sun: Financial picture begins turn-around."

Melton was firmly convinced that the company would survive. Employees were beginning to believe him. Persuading the public, and especially the distrustful media, was more difficult, however. Following the press conference of February 26, one Dallas newspaper hired two analysts to review financial statements. Melton gave the newspaper permission to come on-site to look at the books. The story that resulted was headlined, "Blue Cross Wages Battle to Remain Solvent," and was primarily many inches of newsprint stating the obvious but slanted toward the negative. It was picked up on newswires and ended up in newspapers across the state. Melton felt betrayed by the coverage. One year later when the newspaper again requested permission to come on-site to inspect the books, Melton refused.

As the company focused on the recovery plan, the media attention continued throughout 1982. To round out the senior management team, Melton hired Jeffery P. Langmead as senior vice president for claims effective April 2. In June Aune retired, leaving Melton and the five senior vice presidents as the executive team.

The marketplace's confidence had eroded. The company had bid on several former groups, and, though it was the low bidder, the groups elected not to return. Several major accounts were lost, and membership took a significant dip, but during the year several advances were made.

On November 1 TotalCare, a new individual comprehensive health and life insurance product, was released to the market. This product offered more comprehensive benefits than the company's Texas Trail Blazer individual policy. A home office telephone sales and service center was set up to sell the product as well as a small group product. It was marketed primarily through mailouts and on the phone.

By the end of the year, the marketplace's attitude toward the company changed favorably, as evidenced in November when, for the first time since 1981, the number of contracts enrolled exceeded the cancellations received.

Other hopeful signs were evident. To improve service to important national accounts, the company created a dedicated unit in Customer Service and, to help staff rate more accurately, it implemented a new rating monitoring system. Utilization trends were looking more favorable, and it was hoped that with the hospital price cap and UCR implementation, finances would improve. Claims inventory and error rates were down.

Several cost containment initiatives were introduced, including an ambulatory surgery program that promoted surgery in the doctor's office when medically appropriate. The company adopted a more stringent stance with hospitals on over-utilization and stood firm against hospitals that did not cooperate, canceling the Member Hospital contracts of two hospitals. Because the Alamo Health Care Plan was not a successful venture and was draining resources, the company withdrew from the plan at the end of 1982.

In September Melton told the board that the hospital price cap had served its purpose. He recommended that the cap be discontinued on September 21 but that "hard, tough" negotiations with each hospital continue, to be monitored by himself.

In early 1983, as year-end 1982 figures came into focus, Melton prepared for yet another round of media activity with the filing of financial statements with the State Board of Insurance. On Monday morning, February 28, as the corporate annual statements were being delivered to the State Board of Insurance, a press release was once again simultaneously delivered to board members, the news media and employees across the state.

The news was good: At year-end 1982, the company posted a $9.3 million loss. The statement emphasized that this loss was better than expected (and certainly better than the $36.1 million loss in 1981 or the $47.3 million loss in 1980). That amounted to a 74 percent reduction in losses from 1981. Surplus was up to $26.9 million.

Soon, the headlines across the state reflected the optimism of the recovered company. "Blue Cross of Texas gains strength" headlined the *Dallas Morning News,* and the *Houston Chronicle* asserted: "Melton's medicine may cure the ills of Blue Cross."

In May several significant events indicated the company was winning the recovery war. April had been the company's best month ever for claims processing with an average 6.2 day turnaround. Claims inventory was down to seventy-nine thousand. State Board examiners who had been in-house since 1981 were recalled to Austin, indicating confidence in the company's progress. And company leaders finally had a contract in hand for the sale and leaseback of the Richardson building. The deal would eventually close in August and enhance the cash position.

By June, business was almost back to normal. In his report to the board that month, Melton announced a $2.9 million gain for the month of

May. The board spontaneously burst into a hearty round of applause. The corner had been turned. The company had been saved.

A new advertising campaign premiered the next month, the first in two and one-half years, that reflected the new enthusiasm, pronouncing Blue Cross and Blue Shield of Texas as "The Health Care Company You Can Feel Good About."

With recovery in hand, the company began to push more assertively in the marketplace in 1983. A major change in marketing strategy was announced. Beginning July 1 the company allowed selected independent agents and brokers, in addition to the company's internal sales force, to market Blue Cross and Blue Shield of Texas products. This was no small culture change. From the beginning the company had its own sales force and prided itself on its difference from commercial competitors. But now, marketplace realties demanded a change. With the theme, "On Our Way," the broker program was kicked off in May with a seminar at the home office.

In August Melton announced to employees that the month's sales were the best in more than two years. The new sales figures also showed an encouraging trend: many groups that had dropped Blue Cross and Blue Shield coverage in the early 1980s were returning.

Advantage I, a small group program for employers of ten to twenty-four employees, was introduced. (It was revised in 1985 as Advantage II.) Most group policies were enhanced to cover cornea, liver, kidney, heart and heart-lung transplants, reflecting advancing medical technology.

Cost containment began to enter a new era. Before, the company depended on the voluntary cooperation of members and health care providers to contain costs. By now, however, cost containment was beginning to be a matter of built-in financial incentives and disincentives for the member. A new cost-containment package included day surgery and mandated second opinion surgery before elective surgery, pre-admission testing, no weekend admission unless an emergency, home health care, hospice care, generic drugs, and extended care facilities. The next step in cost containment, pre-admission certification, which would certify in-patient admissions before the patient was admitted, was being developed and would be introduced later.

Managing information systems

The conversion of the systems other than the claims processing system was delayed because of the problems of the 1980 conversion. The company began to prepare for converting membership and billing records to the more automated system to be implemented on June 1, 1983. Lessons well learned in the data processing conversion contributed to a successful and relatively trouble-free conversion.

The next major systems conversion was the Medicare system. Pascasio was due to retire on March 1, 1983, but remained with the company to manage the conversion. The conversion was scheduled for May 1984 and, like the other recent conversions, was very successful. Pascasio retired on May 31 with the successful conversion behind him. The board was especially complimentary of Raymond Hunter's role in managing the conversion. In December 1984 he was named a senior vice president. Hunter joined the company in 1967 in the information systems area and transferred employment to EDS in 1979, one of many company employees transferred because of the data processing contract. He rejoined the company in 1980.

Hunter advised the board in early 1985 that the contract with EDS would expire in 1988 and that they needed to be thinking if the function should stay with a vendor or be brought inside.

The increasing financial and operational strength paved the way for several changes within the company.

What could have been the most radical change and yet was not noticed by most employees was the company's relationship with the Blue Cross and Blue Shield Association (BCBSA). In the mid-1980s, that relationship became strained.

In July 1983 Melton informed the executive committee of BCBSA's Long-Term Business Strategy, which was an attempt of the Association to centralize more control. In certain areas, this would diminish control of local boards of directors. This provoked much discussion within the System of Plans, including Texas. Melton vigorously opposed the strategy, and for years the BCBSA and Melton tugged at each other over how much the System should be centralized or decentralized. Melton seriously considered the possibility of the company leaving the System and took steps to protect the name and service marks. Group Hospital Service, Inc., was renamed Blue Cross and Blue Shield of Texas, Inc., in 1984 (the state approved the name change in December 1983) to establish the name and service marks in Texas as well as to send a message to BCBSA that the Texas Plan intended to stay in control of its own destiny. However, the concerns over the Long-Term Business Strategy finally faded and relationships improved.

Melton had become active on the national level of the Blue Cross and Blue Shield System. He served the Federal Employee Program's (FEP) board of managers from 1984 to 1989, the FEP finance subcommittee from 1984 to 1986 and the FEP audit subcommittee in 1988 and 1989.

While this drama was playing out in the executive offices, the culture of everyday work life shifted. A July 1984 memo to employees announced the wellness program, Healthworks (renamed Motiva in 1994). It had existed since 1980 in the Public Information Department, primarily as a health promotion function. In 1984 it was enhanced to focus on stress management, nutrition counseling, weight control, exercise, and smoking cessation. In the first part of the program, employees could undergo a blood test, fitness evaluation and a health risk appraisal. Programs were then offered to help employees improve their health. The company had enrolled a large school district in the state, and their proposal included assistance in setting up a wellness program for employees. As was often the case, Blue Cross and Blue Shield of Texas employees were guinea pigs for new programs piloted in-house and then taken to the marketplace.

Healthworks would eventually find a home in a modern fitness center, but, in the beginning days, exercise classes were held in the east lobby and in the third floor executive dining room. "Now you can hardly walk through the office," noted *Advance* magazine, "without tripping over somebody's exercise pad."[8] The wellness movement also brought a new fashion statement to the company: during breaks employees in business suits and skirts would don athletic shoes.

Even for those less athletically inclined, business dress was becoming more casual. In May 1985 each Friday was designated as denim day when employees could dress more casually.

Big changes were happening in Medicare during this era. In 1983 Medicare mandated paying hospital claims with the Diagnosis Related Group (DRG) method which determined cost by diagnosis rather than by cost reimbursement. In 1984 the Health Care Financing Administration instituted the Participating Physician Program. Prior to the program, physicians could choose whether to accept an assignment on a claim-by-claim basis. In the new program, physicians could sign agreements that bound them to accept assignments on all Medicare claims. (As the program moved forward in later years, physicians were limited in the amount they could charge Medicare patients on non-assigned claims.) For the first time, the Medicare division published a participating physician directory.

In October 1984 the UB-82 claim form was implemented after many years of work by a consortium of BCBSA, commercial insurers, government entities and others so that all hospital claims (whether for Blue Cross, Medicare, Medicaid or other third-party payers) could be filed on one form. The issue had first been raised in 1968 with the first national committee formed in 1975.

In July 1985 Medicare made a massive conversion to a new required national procedure code system—HCPCS—which employed twenty thousand procedure codes instead of the former seventy-five hundred codes in processing Medicare claims. In September of that year, Medicare employees got a new home when the division moved from the leased Brookriver location to renovated quarters in the north building at the home office.

Year-end 1983 financial figures showed a solid gain of $13.7 million. A year later, at year-end 1984, the news was exceedingly good. The company posted a gain of $27 million in 1984—the most profitable year in the company's history. Melton quickly took advantage of the improved financials to begin the work of establishing a 401(k) tax deferral plan for employees, called the Money Matcher plan.

With the company fully recovered financially and operationally, Melton decided it was time to turn over the reins of the presidency. He was better suited, he thought, to being a troubleshooter. He announced to the board that he wished to retire on April 30, 1985.

To take his place, he recommended William P. Daves, former chairman of the State Board of Insurance. Melton agreed to stay on as chairman of the board, replacing John Justin, Jr. who would step down as chairman. On April 26 the board approved the appointments and also named Justin chairman emeritus of the board.

Daves quietly assumed office on May 1 and just as quietly left a month later. The match between Daves and the company was not a good one. On June 1 Melton returned to his familiar post as president and CEO, and Bill Collins was named chairman of the board.

Early managed care

In the mid-1980s a new term was being used in health care circles. "Managed care" was replacing the well-worn term, "cost containment." Melton noted that the health care marketplace was being altered by the spread of health maintenance organizations (HMO) and preferred provider organizations (PPO) and that the new arrangements were drastically altering relationships. "Our biggest competitors are rapidly becoming hospitals and physicians," he said at the time. And he knew that would change the company. "We've got to be able to deliver to the public what they want. We're going to push very hard on ways to stabilize the cost of medical care."[9]

One way this new environment affected the company was at the board of directors level. Both the TMA and the THA's highest elected officials had seats on the board as ex-officio members. The bylaws were revised to remove these honorary positions, a sign of shifting relationships.

PPOs were most popular with the market, but, in Texas, insurance laws did not allow contracting for physician services. A provision of Chapter 20 of the insurance code, under which the company operated, specifically prohibited contracting for physician services. In 1986 the State Board of Insurance adopted new rules, which allowed for the formation of PPOs by commercial carriers. However, PPO activity was not yet great, so company leaders decided it was not the appropriate time to develop one. (Later in 1988 company leaders worked to introduce legislation in Texas that would amend Chapter 20 and allow the Texas Plan to sign contracts with physicians and form a PPO. The bill passed in 1989.)

Until the company could develop a full-fledged PPO, it proceeded with the creation of a managed care product that stopped short of actually contracting for services. On September 1, 1986, TexasCare hit the market. It included various early managed care features such as pre-certification, pre-admission testing, discharge planning, large case management, extended care coverage, second opinion surgery, day surgery, private-duty nursing, and preventive care. (In 1987 a small group version of the product—TexasCare 24—was released.)

At approximately the same time, the company introduced its first prescription drug program card, which made it possible for subscribers to purchase prescriptions with a simple co-payment. It was administered through an agreement with Blue Cross and Blue Shield of Western New York, which processed claims and provided a ready-made national network of pharmacies. Generic drugs were available at lower co-payments.

Adding to the company's increasing managed care mix was an HMO. The company reached an agreement in September 1985 with Blue Cross and Blue Shield of New Mexico to operate a joint venture HMO in El Paso, giving the company experience in operating an HMO. The joint venture was named Rio Grande Choice Health Plan. Rio Grande received its license to do business on March 30, 1987, and began marketing activities. In 1988 the company purchased the New Mexico Plan's share of the HMO, which had been renamed Rio Grande HMO, Inc., and moved its domicile from New Mexico to Texas.

In late 1986 another acronym entered the company vernacular: TPA (third party administrator). The company formed a TPA called HealthCare Benefits, Inc. A TPA worked with groups that self-funded their benefit plans, acting as a third party to process claims and purchase various service components of a group benefit plan.

In late 1986 and early 1987, the company began putting together what became the foundation for later physician networks. The Texas Professional Payment Plan (or PPP for short) was a simple agreement where physicians agreed to file claims for the member and accept the company's Reasonable Charge amount as the full payment. They also agreed to not balance-bill the patient. This was an important step in the company's marketing strategy. UCR had been a successful payment mechanism, but, if the physician's charge was more than the UCR amount, the patient was left responsible for the unpaid balance. Physician directories, then still a rarity in the pre-managed care age, were distributed to groups in October 1987.

Melton put Rogers K. Coleman, M.D., in charge of constructing the PPP. Coleman was formerly an associate medical director and was promoted to vice president/medical director in 1986. In May 1987 solicitation for physicians began, and the program was implemented on September 1.

The late 1980s also saw several significant pieces of federal legislation which affected business. In 1985 the Consolidated Omnibus Budget Reconciliation Act (COBRA) passed, which provided for continuation of coverage for terminated employees and dependents on groups with twenty or more employees. In 1986 Blue Cross and Blue Shield Plans lost their tax-exempt status as a part of federal tax legislation. Also that year, federal law required that alcoholism be treated as any other illness.

On January 7, 1986, employees got a big surprise. Upon Melton's recommendation the board approved a surprise bonus for employees, the amount based on years of service. The bonus was in appreciation for employees' loyalty and hard work during the difficult times of the early 1980s and their contributions in recent years, which resulted in the company's return to a viable, profitable position.

In late 1986 a new "employee" began making rounds throughout the company. The "mailmobile" was an automated cart that ran on an invisible chemical trail in the carpet, programmed to stop at selected spots. At first it was a novelty to see a machine rove through the building with no attendant, but employees quickly got used to it. (One cart even began sporting a simulated employee ID badge that some industrious employee fashioned.)

At the end of the year, in December, division managers were all made vice presidents.

In August 1987 the executive committee took action to protect the employee retirement funds by moving the company pension fund to an outside trustee. The funds had previously been co-mingled with company funds and conceivably could have been lost in a dire financial situation.

In March 1988 the life data processing system was transferred inhouse. Then, on October 11 the regular business health claims processing system was also brought in-house. This was the final conversion to in-house systems. Now, for the first time in nearly ten years, critical data processing functions were again fully under the ownership and control of the company. In addition, the conversions had gone very smoothly.

Preparing for a new era

Melton surprised the company in September 1988 by announcing that the board had named Coleman as executive vice president, effective October 1. Coleman himself was surprised that he had been selected as Melton's successor-elect.

"It shocked me," Coleman recalled. "I had no idea that I was in the running, and I had never even had any aspirations for the job."

There were no guarantees, however, Melton told Coleman. If he didn't work out as executive vice president, he wouldn't be named president. On the day Coleman received the news from Melton, he told his wife Mary Lou, "I probably won't make it, so prepare for us to go hunt something else to do. But we'll give it a try."[10]

As soon as Coleman was named EVP, the rate of change in the company accelerated.

Melton's first assignment for Coleman was to coordinate a process to manage the unbundling of charges on claims. Some physicians had discovered that submitting separate charges for each individual component of a service, instead of submitting one all-encompassing fee for the service, would result in higher payment. The automated claims payment system had to be reconfigured to be able to properly re-bundle these charges to pay the series of services more accurately. The project was completed and the system activated by January 1990.

On December 15, 1989, the board elected Coleman chief operating officer in addition to his title of executive vice president, a vote of confidence in the direction the company had taken.

In late 1989 Coleman announced that the state was interested in developing a special insurance pool for high-risk individuals so that people with a serious illness could purchase health insurance. Coleman was selected for the board of the Texas Health Insurance Risk Pool. The board's task was to develop a plan of operation to give to the State Board of Insurance. In December 1990 Coleman announced that the Texas Plan had been chosen as the program's administrator, but the state failed to fund the program, and it lay dormant for several years. Eventually, though, it fulfilled its mission and provided health insurance to those unable to purchase it because of health status.

In April 1990 it was announced that the company was awarded the bid for the Medicare Common Working File project. The Texas Plan was one of two Plans in the nation chosen to design and implement an experimental regional database used to pay claims in the southwest region of the country.

In June 1990 a new individual health insurance policy was released to the marketplace. Select 2000 replaced TotalCare, which had been taken off the market earlier. Select 2000 was an individual product aimed at the small business market. It was sold as a payroll deduction product and marketed through brokers.

Company growth resulted in employee growth, which was again squeezing space, a familiar situation throughout the history of the company. Employees and departments began to be moved into leased or purchased buildings along Sherman Street near the Richardson headquarters. In 1990 the company purchased additional land and a building in Denison to accommodate the successful growth of Medicare operations in that city.

At the board meeting on December 14, 1990, Melton announced his retirement as of the end of the month. Being primarily a financial man, he was pleased to report to the board that 1990 looked to be an excellent financial year, and once again he wanted to reward employees. Melton recommended another employee bonus, and the board approved.

At the same meeting, Coleman was elected president and chief executive officer, effective January 1, 1991.

Melton left the company quietly and distanced himself from too many overt accolades, for he was at heart a private man who felt he was just doing his job for the company. But for those employees who had toughed out the early 1980s and then saw the company rebound stronger than before, largely because of the leadership of one man, it was difficult not to offer accolades.

Employees, however, didn't have long to linger in fond memories of Melton. At the same board meeting that ratified Melton's retirement and Coleman's ascension to the company's highest staff office, there was a small piece of news that would drastically change the scope of company operations. Two major accounts—one existing longtime group and one large prospective national account—were asking for a provider network, something the company didn't have. To keep the one account and capture the other, the company would have to develop a network of physicians and hospitals across the wide expanse of Texas and do it in just one year.

The new era had begun even before Coleman sat down in the president's chair.

13 | 1991-1998: Facing the Future

*"Improving our operations and pursuing
new ventures are not optional. We
must move forward."*
Rogers K. Coleman, M.D.

The organization Rogers K. Coleman, M.D., inherited as he settled into his new role as president was one with a rich history of serving Texans. That heritage, Coleman knew, provided significant advantages in the health care marketplace. It also provided impediments.

The company's history of having close economic and political ties with Texas hospitals and doctors actually was a disadvantage. "In the distant past," Coleman wrote in an article for the employee magazine, "the medical care system was controlled by doctors and hospitals, and our close relationship was an advantage. Over the past several years, the medical care system increasingly has come to be controlled by payers— government- and employee-sponsored groups. The system has changed from being provider-driven to payer-driven, and our heritage has made it hard for us to shed our historic image. The key to our future success lies in forging a new partnership between payers and providers. This is a new role as facilitator/intermediary. Thomas Paine said, 'Those who are planning for posterity should remember that virtue is not inherited.'"[1]

It was a new age in health care. The company had to face it and change dramatically. Coleman was the person called to lead the process.

Rogers King Coleman was born December 28, 1931, in Palestine, Texas. Since childhood he knew he wanted to be a doctor. His father was a physician, practicing literally until the day he died in 1965. Initially, Coleman intended to do his undergraduate pre-med work at Texas Tech College (now University) in Lubbock, but he met a young woman named Mary Lou Price and she was headed to college at Texas Christian University in Fort Worth. "So like any smitten young man, I immediately changed plans and went to TCU. I've never regretted that decision."[2] They were married in 1951 as Coleman finished his pre-med education at TCU. He then continued his studies at Baylor Medical School in Houston and graduated from there in 1956. After residency training the Coleman family moved to Brownwood, Texas, where he was in private practice from 1958 to 1976 as a family physician. He also served as chief of staff at Brownwood Community Hospital and on its board of trustees.

Despite his love of the profession, he grew weary of being on call twenty-four hours a day. Louis W. Conradt, M.D., medical director of the company in 1975, talked to him about coming to Dallas to join the medical staff. They had met while serving on a committee of the TMA. At first, Coleman said no, but later that year he drove to Dallas to talk with company officials and in February 1976 accepted the position.

"At first I was just looking for a change and really didn't intend on staying long. But the more involved I got in my job, the more interested I became in the issues of health care financing."[3] In 1986 he advanced to medical director, and in 1988 Melton selected him to be executive vice president.

On January 1, 1991, he became the company's top staff leader at a time when the company had to move fast to keep up and maintain its leadership position.

Building a network

Of all the challenges ahead in the next decade, the biggest task was to shift to a more customer-focused position. The 1991 marketing plan visually demonstrated the task by showing an inverted corporate organization chart with the customer, not the executive leadership, on top.

It was clear that customers in Texas were beginning to demand managed care networks. Two bids were expected in-house. One was from a prominent national account. The other was from the State of Texas, a longtime customer of the company. Both required managed care networks. Beyond the needs of these two accounts, it was evident that the time had come to build a network to serve growing market demand.

Building a hospital network was relatively easy—the company had existing contracts with virtually all Texas hospitals, which provided a foundation for negotiating point of service contracts. The company also changed its method of reimbursing hospitals, introducing the Diagnosis

Related Group (DRG) program, helping to usher in managed care with hospitals. (DRGs assigned an average weight to each case to gauge the severity of a condition and the cost of treatment. Hospitals received a predetermined amount for each case, reducing the cost of hospital care.)

Building a physician network, however, was a different story. From the company's beginnings, physician benefits had been carefully designed to allow the physician autonomy and the capability of choosing what to charge patients. Now was the time to talk with physicians across the great expanse of Texas, negotiating contract provisions and payments with Texas' independent-minded physicians. In early 1991 the company hired Ron Atkins, M.D., to lead the process of recruiting physicians for the network.

At the same time as building the network, the company also was reaching out to physicians to join yet another program: ParPlan, which replaced the Professional Payment Plan agreement. ParPlan was similar to the former Professional Payment Plan but with the added advantage of providing direct reimbursement only to participating professionals. (The TMA later sponsored legislation that required insurers to provide direct payment to all physicians, whether participating or not.)

Besides building the actual network, the entire company had to completely re-gear to provide benefits and services in a network/non-network environment. Two individuals were appointed to head the task: Bill Crowley, vice president of Claims, who directed the internal elements of the project (administrative, claims, data processing systems, product development) and newly named vice president of Provider Affairs, Lyn Cypert, who headed the external elements of the project (hospital and facility issues, physicians, pharmacies and suppliers).

A task force was set up of key employees from each division. Virtually no area of the company was unaffected. The list of events that had to take place seemed never-ending: draw up new contracts with myriad health care professionals and facilities, develop information systems, establish responsive customer service capabilities, produce provider directories, and test and retest all systems to make sure everything worked as planned. Benefits would be administered on a network and non-network basis, and procedures had to be established to allow this. Once the network was developed and running, various constituencies of the company would have to be educated on the new managed care environment: providers, suppliers, members, group decision makers and the public at large. Sales literature and enrollment literature would have to be developed and provider directories published. The network and the benefit product would have to be named. (BlueChoice was selected as the name for both.)

A "war room" was set up where staff hovered daily. Regular meetings of all team members led by Crowley's no-nonsense management style ensured the project stayed on track.

Early in the project, Cypert skillfully communicated the essence of the project ahead in one simple visual. He had a slide prepared that showed a turtle with a rocket ship tied to its back, and a hand was reaching forward with a match about to light the rocket. The hand was marked, "Dr. Coleman."

Indeed, the rocket had been launched.

Point of service was a new term that described a managed care program that used a network similar to a health maintenance organization (HMO) but allowed the member to go outside the network for care but at a lower reimbursement. Benefits were richer within the network. Simple copayments paid at the time of service replaced the age-old familiar task of paying the doctor, filing the claim, and waiting for reimbursement. Case managers worked to maintain the quality of health care services while also maintaining cost efficiency. There were two basic versions of the benefit product itself. BlueChoice® Plus was a "gatekeeper" plan that required all care to be managed by a primary care physician. (In 1993 the BlueChoice point of service contract became a preferred provider organization—PPO—contract.) BlueChoice® was a managed health care plan but with no "gatekeeper," so members could go directly to specialists without a referral.

The Texas Plan submitted the bid for the large national account but didn't get the business. However, by the spring of 1992, the company received word that it had won the bid for the State of Texas employees and retirees group, and the program became effective on September 1. This was a major accomplishment, as it also signified the end of very hard work in putting together a statewide network of physicians and hospitals.

Implementing the state program took a massive effort. Staff traveled all across the state holding 1,500 meetings with state agencies to transfer the 100,000 enrollees to the new benefit plan, adding 30,000 to 40,000 new higher education enrollees to the state group, increasing the Austin office to accommodate the enrollment, adding physicians and hospitals to the provider networks, communicating with state group employees, and preparing new simple language benefit booklets for enrollees.

Again, company employees assumed their role of being a laboratory for the new provider network. In July, before the state program became effective in September, the company announced that employees residing in the Dallas, Fort Worth, Austin, San Antonio and Houston network service areas were now covered by the managed care plan.

Besides covering the state group and company employees, BlueChoice was released to the marketplace and was an immediate success. The network was developed in two phases. Phase one involved having the network up in the state's five largest metropolitan areas by early 1992, while phase two called for the network in the next fifteen to twenty largest metropolitan areas by early 1993.

Employees as active partners

Besides all the change in the transition to managed care and the building of the state's largest network of providers, the company was charging forward with change on other fronts.

In 1991 employees had many opportunities to participate actively in the company's direction. Coleman held a series of meetings with employees to communicate progress and plans for the shift to managed care. On October 1 the company instituted an employee suggestion program with a cash award for employees who submitted cost-saving ideas.

On December 13, each employee was given the new mission statement and a strategic plan for the three-year period beginning January 1, 1992. The strategic plan consisted of five broad goals: expand market share, maintain financial solvency, establish a culture that is customer-based and quality focused, be a positive influence on community health, and maintain the company's role as a major player in the Medicare program.

The mission statement was developed at Coleman's request by an employee task force representing all divisions, chaired by Carolyn Colley. The committee members spent months in discussion during 1991 to develop the mission statement, which read:

> We are dedicated to serving our customers through the financing of health care and related benefits services.
>
> We will provide products and services of the highest quality and value with a direct focus on meeting the needs of our customers. We will respond to the customer with promptness, sensitivity, respect, and always with integrity.
>
> We are committed to providing an enjoyable work environment for our employees, our most important resource. We will continually promote teamwork, quality improvement, and excellence in all phases of business.
>
> We will maintain a financially strong, growth-oriented company for the protection of our customers and employees.
>
> Through leadership and innovation, we will meet the challenges of the health care delivery system and serve as many Texans as we can.

The new mission to serve as many Texans as possible meant serving in two distinct arenas. One, of course, was the escalating marketing effort to sell more business. The other was to fulfill the role of good corporate citizen and help underserved markets and provide an important public service function.

One of those underserved markets was the growing number of the uninsured in Texas. While all age sectors of the population were affected, children were especially vulnerable. As a physician, Coleman knew that many children's diseases could be remedied early in life by access to primary health care.

Several other Plans had instituted the Caring for Children Program. The program provided a basic package of health benefits covering primary and preventive outpatient health benefits to children whose families earned too much to qualify for Medicaid but did not earn enough to purchase health insurance. In the spring of 1991, Coleman recommended to the board that a Caring Program be sponsored in Texas, with administrative and operational expenses provided by the company. Craig Jeffery was hired to set up the program. In January 1992 the first twenty-six children were enrolled from Hays (San Marcos) and Comal (New Braunfels) counties. As of December 1998, more than six thousand children had been enrolled, and almost $5.5 million in contributions and support had been received. (In 1997 the Texas Legislature enacted the Texas Healthy Kids Corporation, which provided more comprehensive coverage to indigent children. The Caring for Children Foundation of Texas began to shift its focus to supporting the new Healthy Kids venture.)

Moving closer to the customer

Elevating the customer to the top of the organization required more than building a provider network responsive to the customer. It would eventually require a complete reorganization.

In a memo to senior staff and staff officers on August 31, 1993, Coleman announced a reorganization, stating that the company faced major challenges. He commented that while the company had "emerged from financial trouble, it has been at the expense of growth. Growth is of great importance: it allows us to regain our preeminent position in the market; it helps strengthen reserves; it funds new products; and it provides new opportunities to our employees."[4] This growth was to come through an organization that was less hierarchical and vertical and one that would move the company closer to the customer.

Six business units were established based primarily on geographic territories. This was a major change for the organization. According to Coleman, the geographic business units (GBUs) were set up with the "recognition that the Houston customer has needs distinct from the Tyler customer or the Amarillo customer."[5] GBUs would enable the company to be more responsive to customers and more creative in solving problems. Each unit would be responsible for profit and loss and growth of regular business in its area. The new organization was scheduled to begin implementation on January 1, 1994, though full implementation would be beyond that.

The six GBUs and their initial chief operating officers (COO) were: Houston/Southeast Texas, Darren Rodgers; Northeast Texas, Pat Hemingway Hall; Greater Texas, Alan Gorlewski; West Texas, Bill Worley; Midwest Texas, Larry Bowermon; South Texas, Russ Sanderson. (In 1998 the South Texas GBU was integrated into the Midwest and Southeast GBUs. Also, the rural counties of the Greater Texas GBU were integrated into the GBUs serving metropolitan counties.)

In addition to the GBUs, two strategic business units (SBU) with vice presidents/COOs were set up: Lelia Wright headed up Medicare, and Jackie Hamilton, the Federal Employee Program and HealthCare Benefits, Inc. Key home office functions reported to Raymond Hunter, senior vice president/COO of Core Services.

Upper management had been prepared for this massive change in corporate structure. In 1993 top management received training in "change management" and then attended Quality College to learn the principles of quality processes. Throughout 1994, first managers and then employees at all levels were trained in quality concepts.

Quality improvement teams were set up in each business unit. A recognition program was developed to formally honor employees whose work exemplified quality principles or who developed ideas that substantially improved quality processes and reduced errors. Some rewards were monetary, with the most prestigious quality award, the Beacon Award, presented annually to two employees who have shown exceptional achievement in the quality process.

In early 1994 the company ventured into another state program aimed at helping markets that had difficulty getting health insurance. The company was selected as administrator of the Texas Insurance Purchasing Alliance, a state initiative to provide small businesses (three to fifty employees) with access to affordable health coverage. Employees of alliance members were able to choose coverage from a number of qualified plans. The company served a dual function as administrator of the alliance, and also as a supplier of coverage to small businesses, competing with other carriers.

That same year, company leaders looked beyond the state's southern border for new business opportunities—specifically Mexico. Many hospitals in Texas were already delivering health care to Mexican citizens. In partnership with the Arizona Plan, the Texas Plan formed Arizona/ Texas International, Inc. (ATI) to develop products under the brand of Blue Cross and Blue Shield of Mexico. (ATI bid on and was awarded the license to use the Blue Cross and Blue Shield names and service marks in Mexico.) Mexico was an untapped insurance market with an estimated ninety million consumers. Though the country's health care services were provided largely under a government program, there was discussion that the system ought to be privatized. ATI began looking for an established Mexican private insurance company with which to align to establish the project and minimize risk. In June 1998 the initiative was renamed Arizona/California/Texas International, Inc., when Blue Shield of California became a shareholder.

The site of another strategic venture was within national boundaries. In June 1994 the company announced that the Health Care Financing Administration (HCFA) had awarded the company the contract to process Medicare Part B claims for the state of Maryland, effective January 1, 1995. The Medicare Part B business was being transferred from the Maryland Plan. In Maryland, the company's operations were doing business as TrailBlazer. This new venture was the first major company operation outside of Texas. (In 1998 an actual subsidiary was formed to do the business—TrailBlazer Health Enterprises, LLC.)

This first foray outside state bounderies positioned the company to gain more Medicare contracts from the federal government and to increase service to more beneficiaries of the program. The company had long excelled in the Medicare program. It had been Texas' original Medicare contractor in 1966 when the massive federal program began. Over the years new responsibilities were awarded to the company: as Region 6 Intermediary for End Stage Renal Disease claims, the Common Working File Host Site for the Southwest Sector and the National CWF Beta Site.

In 1997 HCFA awarded the Texas Plan the contract to expand Part B operations for beneficiaries in the District of Columbia, Arlington and Fairfax counties as well as the city of Alexandria in northern Virginia, Prince Georges and Montgomery counties in Maryland, and the state of Delaware. This expansion made the company one of the largest Medicare contractors in the nation.

In November 1995 the company became the Medicare Part A intermediary for New Mexico and Colorado. Just after that announcement was made, HCFA awarded the company another large contract—to serve as intermediary for freestanding rural health clinics in Arkansas, Colorado, Louisiana, Montana, New Mexico, North Dakota, Oklahoma, South Dakota, Texas, Utah and Wyoming. In 1997 the company was awarded the contract for processing Oklahoma claims on the Florida Shared System.

By the end of the 1990s, TrailBlazer served more than 3.7 million Medicare beneficiaries in seven states.

As the company's base of markets and customers expanded, so did its technological expertise. The company had begun Provider Automation in the 1970s, and hospitals and physicians slowly began to file claims electronically. By the mid 1990s, more than 70 percent of the company's total claims were paperless. The company used this expertise to provide a worthy service for the health care community—the Texas Health Information Network℠ was unveiled at a press conference in Austin on November 15, 1994. The network was an electronic clearinghouse where physicians, hospitals and other providers could file patient claims to multiple insurance companies and government benefit programs. The Texas Plan had been involved in electronic claims for fourteen years, and this was a major leadership advance to use its expertise to benefit everyone. The company developed the program in conjunction with the TMA and the THA.

Employee life

Throughout the 1990s, a number of changes in the company affected the workaday world of employees.

Even with advancing electronic communications, the insurance business produced paperwork—and lots of it. In February 1991 the company, with the cooperation of its employees, put its paper refuse to good work with a large-scale corporate recycling program. In the first eighteen days of the program, a daily average of 4,857 pounds of paper were sold.

With a sensitivity to the effects of smoking on health, the company made its home office building a non-smoking facility on January 1, 1992, causing a record number of employees to enroll in Healthworks' smoking cessation classes.

As the company embraced teamwork as a quality measure, it sought ways to increase communication and collaboration in an atmosphere of mutual respect. Responding to a suggestion from Sam Schaal (in the employee suggestion program), the company made the background color of badges the same for all employees in September 1994. Previously, the background color signified which of three tiers (executive, managerial and professional, clerical and technical) one belonged. Coleman summed up this improvement this way, "We want to make teamwork visible in all aspects of our company and begin to remove any real or perceived obstacles to that objective." [6]

Business environments of the 1990s were becoming more comfortable and casual places in which to work, with companies allowing employees to wear business casual attire. Coleman announced a revised dress code on February 14, 1995, providing the opportunity for employees to dress daily in casual business wear.

Another pioneering move

Change had become the order of the day. "Improving our operations and pursuing new ventures are not optional," Coleman told employees in a 1995 memo. "We must move forward."[7] The change in the company was dizzying at times, but Coleman was about to push the organization forward into an even more radical change.

One of the real needs was a more advanced information system. Keeping up-to-date with the latest technology was one of the company's keys to success, and without leading-edge systems, the company's future was bleak. As Coleman related, "Even though we were in love with our regular business claims system, it was an old system. It had not had any significant upgrades, and we needed more sophisticated systems."[8] To invest in these systems and other efficiencies necessary for growth required additional capital. Additional capital required a much larger company.

Coleman was about to suggest a change that was bold for a company that prided itself in its Lone Star roots. The chronology of events that led to this bold move shows the logic and common sense of those working toward a more secure and successful future for the company.

In a report to the board on June 30, 1995, Coleman indicated that the company was meeting with a number of other Blue Cross and Blue Shield Plans to explore mutual interests, common processes and ways to improve efficiency. Three months later the Board gave its approval for the company to proceed with nonbinding discussions to align with another Plan. On July 21 employees received a memo from Coleman noting that the company was having discussions with several other Blue Plans. He explained that the company was "exploring the potential for various strategic alliances up to and including the possibility of a merger." He stated simply, "The reason we would enter a strategic alliance would be to strengthen our presence in the marketplace, which would help us grow and prosper as a company."[9]

In November, officers and key directors began a process of refining strategic goals. The process produced the 1996 Strategic Plan, which Coleman presented to the board in December. The plan identified five "strategic drivers" to help the company retain leadership in the health benefits business. The drivers mandated that the company: establish a significant HMO presence in Texas; increase market share; transform business processes, management practices, motivation systems and information systems; develop partnering capabilities; and develop an efficient and flexible distribution system.

Several primary strategies to accomplish these goals were established. One of these was to consider partnership opportunities, including alliances, partnerships, acquisitions, joint ventures and other forms of collaboration.

Early in 1996 employees received the strategic plan in the form of a foldout map—"The Roadmap to Transformation: The 1996 Strategic Plan." The theme of "Lighting the Paths to Our Future Success" was illustrated with a glowing lantern, patterned (of course) after a Coleman brand lantern.

The framework for success was now in place. Next, the company's leadership was to make the pioneering move that was received with mixed emotions by many employees. On January 19 and 20 of 1996, officers from the Texas and Illinois Plans met to discuss an alliance. They notified their respective boards of directors of the recommendation to seek board approval for an alliance with the intent to merge.

On January 29, 1996, Coleman announced to employees: "We have agreed to form an affiliation with Blue Cross and Blue Shield of Illinois to combine operations with an eye toward merger." The strength of the combined plans was impressive. "Between them, the Plans presently provide health care coverage to approximately 3.8 million people, have annual revenues of nearly $6 billion and total reserves of over $1 billion."[10] In deciding to partner with Blue Cross and Blue Shield of Illinois, the company had validated the Illinois Plan's strength in several key elements of an ideal partnering candidate: similar corporate values, advanced technology infrastructure, comprehensive managed care product line, national account service capability, geographic diversity and strong financial standing.

On January 30 the two Plans simultaneously issued a joint press release in Dallas and Chicago. Standard and Poor's subsequently released its favorable review of the prospective merger.

On April 26 the board approved a resolution to proceed with the Illinois Plan, and on May 31 the officers of both the Texas and Illinois Plans met in Chicago where the interim organizational structure was presented. The proposed new board would have ten members from Illinois, including Illinois Plan President Ray McCaskey, and six from Texas, including Coleman.

The six initial board spots to be held by Texas directors on the Health Care Service Corporation (HCSC) board were to be filled by Coleman,

Milton Carroll, Tieman H. "Skipper" Dippel, Jr., Ray Farabee, Jack A. Griggs and James L. Jones. HCSC officers Theodore E. Desch, Joanne M. Rounds, Michael F. Seibold and Sherman M. Wolff were elected senior vice presidents of the Texas Plan, effective July 1. They joined four Texas senior vice presidents (Raymond Hunter, Mike Lewis, Ross Snyder and Lelia Wright) who, in turn, were elected senior vice presidents of the Illinois Plan.

On July 10 the company filed the Texas-Illinois Plan merger documents with the Texas Department of Insurance. Shortly after the filing, the Texas Attorney General's office requested information about the merger plans of the two companies. In a message to the company, Coleman expressed optimism about the merger: "As many of you know, I'm a born optimist. So, it shouldn't surprise you that I feel very good about our pending consolidation with the Illinois Plan. Not only do I look forward to a boom in our business, but I am excited about the tremendous opportunities that each of us will have."[11]

But the Texas attorney general's office had other ideas about the merger.

On November 14 the attorney general filed a lawsuit in Travis County District Court seeking to block the proposed merger between the Texas and Illinois plans. The suit contended that the Texas Plan was a charity and its assets were a charitable trust owned by the people of the state of Texas. It was also the attorney general's position that no Texas law allowed the Texas Plan as a not-for-profit organization to merge into a mutual insurance company like HCSC.

It was becoming clear that the company's bold move toward merger was not going to be as easy to accomplish as hoped.

Meeting customers' needs

In addition to the hard work and the excitement associated with the anticipated merger, the company was making great strides in meeting customers' needs with a growing number of innovative products and services.

A number of HMO programs were developed. HMO Blue® became the marketing name for the wholly owned subsidiary, Rio Grande HMO, Inc., formed in 1987 in El Paso. In the mid-1990s it was expanded into several of Texas' major cities, operating under the name HMO Blue:

• HMO Blue, Southeast Texas, was launched in the Houston and Beaumont areas in April 1994.

• HMO Blue, DFW Metroplex (later renamed Northeast Texas), was also established in April 1994 in the Dallas-Fort Worth area.

• HMO Blue, Central Texas, began in September 1994, serving

Austin, Waco and San Antonio.

* HMO Blue, South Texas, began in Corpus Christi in November 1995.

In two areas of the state, two other HMOs were formed through joint ventures with hospitals:

* West Texas Health Plans, L.C., began in September 1995, doing business as HMO Blue, West Texas, serving the Lubbock and Amarillo areas.

* Mid-Con Health Plans, L. C., began in November 1995, doing business as HMO Blue, SouthWest Texas, serving the San Angelo, Midland, Odessa and Abilene areas.

* HMO Blue Options was established as a HMO-based, point-of-service program available in selected service areas.

The success of HMO Blue helped garner several important Medicaid contracts. In 1996 HMO Blue was awarded Medicaid contracts in the Bexar, Lubbock, Travis and Tarrant county service areas. Harris, Brazoria, Fort Bend, Galveston, Montgomery and Waller counties were added as service areas in 1997. Harris County was also the site of a specialized Medicaid program for chronically ill beneficiaries. (To date, the company's various Medicaid operations serve thirty-five Texas counties with responsibility for over fifty-nine thousand members.)

By the mid-1990s the company portfolio did not just expand, but actually exploded with a plethora of products and services including employee benefit programs, individual health, fee for service plans, HMOs, PPOs, long-term care plans and medical savings accounts.

The company was now in the business of providing unique products to match unique customer needs, giving the customer a product designed to exacting specifications.

The company's public service initiatives also expanded. In 1997 the company launched the Care Van Program within the Caring for Children Foundation. It employed a team of vans that visited schools, churches, shopping centers, restaurants, apartment complexes, recreational parks —wherever kids gathered. Immunizations were provided free of charge and given by volunteer nurses.

In the same year the company fulfilled the promise of obtaining new systems in the move toward merger. Even though the merger was still on hold, the two Plans forged alliances in key areas, and the Texas Plan began converting to the Illinois Plan's Blue Chip system. The Blue Chip system was a highly sophisticated on-line, real-time claims and customer service system. It was integrated with electronic imaging technology that enabled paper claims and customer correspondence to be scanned. With this technology customer service representatives working in full service units (FSUs) were able to access claims and correspondence instantly on screen. Both claims and customer service operations were included in an FSU, allowing a customer to receive information from one location about coverage, claims status, provider networks and most other service issues.

The company also converted the regular business system to Illinois' Blue Chip system, and the payroll and human resources system (in both Illinois and Texas) to the PeopleSoft system.

In 1997 the Texas and Illinois Plans combined their FEP claims and customer service functions in Abilene to handle the program's administrative and customer service operations. (Remaining in the home office in Richardson were FEP's system/network operations and marketing staffs.) FEP initiatives were greatly enhanced by converting to the Illinois Blue Chip system. To manage the conversion, the company trained two hundred Abilene employees.

The FEP program had long been a solid jewel in the company crown. In 1998 the Texas FEP program achieved the third largest net gain (9,116 PPO members) among FEP programs in other Plans. Enrollment gains were significant between 1991 and 1998. In 1991, 181,582 members were enrolled, increasing to 219,181 in 1998.

Other functions were also deployed to other sites. In May 1997 the company announced that a second full service claims and customer service center would open in Marshall. In August the company announced that a third claims and customer service center would be opened in Wichita Falls.

During all this intense activity, employees paused to pay homage to a past company leader. Former president Tom Beauchamp had died March 19, 1998, at age 84.

Path cleared for merger

After almost three years of working toward the merger, the court finally ruled in favor of the company in the lawsuit brought by the attorney general to block the merger. On February 12, 1998, Travis County District Judge Joseph H. Hart ruled that the merger could take place under Texas law because the Texas Plan was not a charity and the Illinois Plan was a not-for-profit organization. The court further ruled that the attorney general would have to pay the Texas Plan's attorneys' fees. The court's decision was the key development in clearing the pathway for the merger.

On September 17 the Texas attorney general reached an agreement with the company and withdrew objections to the merger. The agreement stipulated that the Texas Plan would donate $10 million over five to ten years to the Texas Healthy Kids Corporation. (Under the agreement, the attorney general could appeal only that portion of Judge Hart's February ruling that the Texas Plan was not a charity, but this would not stop the merger from happening. If the attorney general ultimately prevailed upon appeal, the agreement provided that the merged Texas-Illinois Plan would pay the state of Texas $350 million plus 5 percent interest over twenty years to a charitable trust.)

The next step toward the merger was the approval of both the Texas and Illinois departments of insurance as well as formal approval from the boards of directors of both Plans. All of these were obtained in November and December.

So on December 31, 1998, the Texas and Illinois Plans became one company: Health Care Service Corporation, a Mutual Legal Reserve Company (HCSC). In Texas the company would operate as Blue Cross and Blue Shield of Texas, a division of HCSC. In an agreed-upon shared leadership arrangement, Coleman continued his role as president of the (now called) Texas Division, and he also became chairman of the board for HCSC. McCaskey remained the Illinois Division president and also continued as president and CEO of HCSC.

The new company was larger, stronger, and better able to compete in an environment of tough commercial competitors that were large and well financed. The merged company had a year-end 1998 revenue of $8.5 billion and 5.8 million members. The combined Texas and Illinois markets were promising, with thirty-one million total residents in the two states, comprising about one-eighth of the U.S. population. The potential for savings was great, and it was expected that the combined Plans would yield about $100 million in savings over the first three years of its merged existence.

As employees entered the new year of 1999, good news arrived in January as the Texas Division celebrated the milestone of two million members. There had been many company accomplishments during the Coleman era, and one of the most important was the turnaround in membership. "The service improvements provided by the implementation of Blue Chip combined with our broad provider network positioned us as the managed care company of choice," said Pat Hemingway Hall, executive vice president and COO, Texas Division, in a message to employees about the possibilities of future growth.[12] As the new year progressed, the leadership and employees of both Plans focused on shared strengths, merging the best practices and strategies of two large, strong and progressive Plans.

The merger was but another pioneering step for a company with a pioneering history. The Texas and Illinois Plans were now on the vanguard of the Blue Cross and Blue Shield System as a new "Super Blue" regional Plan.

In some ways the merger marked the end of the Texas Plan as a single, autonomous entity. But the end of one story, Coleman noted, has now become the beginning of another. "Our 70 years of service to the people of Texas is not just our past. It also is prologue to the future of our company. As T.S. Eliot has said, 'What we call a beginning is often the end and to make an end is to make a beginning—the end is where we start from.'"[13]

The story of the new regional Health Care Service Corporation, a stronger and more progressive enterprise poised to meet the future of health care head on, is just beginning.

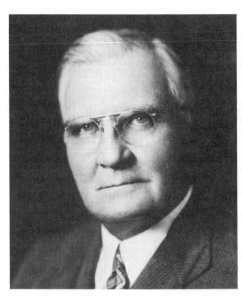

Justin Ford Kimball, the father of group
hospitalization

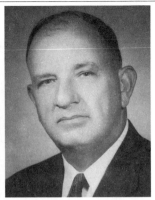

Bryce Twitty, the enthusiastic
promoter of the idea

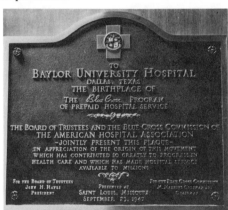

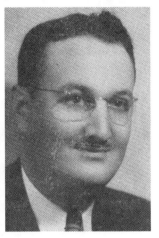

Lawrence Payne, the Baylor
Plan's first employee

Baylor Hospital was officially
recognized as the birthplace of the
national Blue Cross movement in 1947.

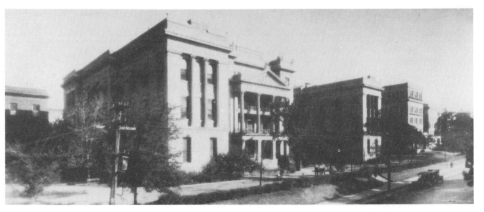

Baylor University Hospital in the 1920s

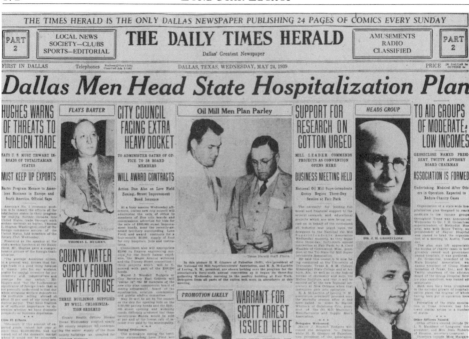

The incorporation of GHS provided the banner headline in the local (second) section of the May 24, 1939, evening newspaper in Dallas. (Collection of the Texas/Dallas History and Archives Division, Dallas Public Library.)

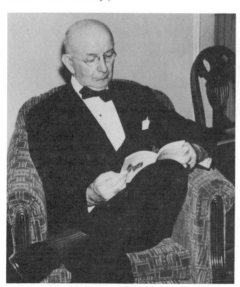

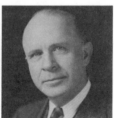

L.N. Markham, M.D.,
vice president

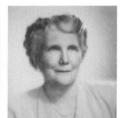

Josie Roberts,
secretary-treasurer

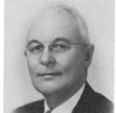

J.H. Groseclose, the first board president

C.E. Hunt

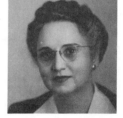

Margaret Hales Rose

The incorporators of GHS – Not pictured are Ara Davis and Martha Roberson

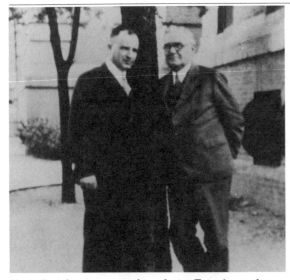

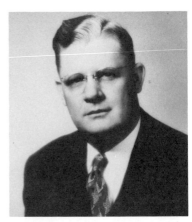

Phil Overton, author of the enabling legislation

Kimball, right, was a consultant during Twitty's tumultuous year as administrator. Kimball was the second administrator of GHS.

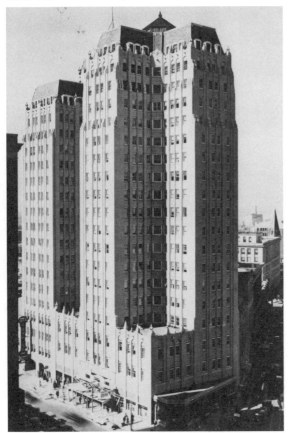

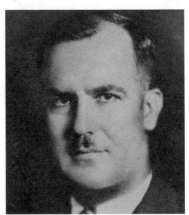

Lucius R. Wilson, M.D., board president for a few months during Groseclose's illness

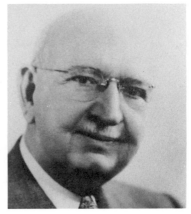

A small suite in Cary's Medical Arts Building was GHS's first location from 1939 to 1940.

E.H. Cary, M.D., board president following Groseclose's death

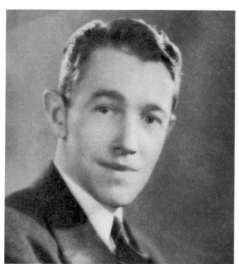

Walter McBee before he came to Texas

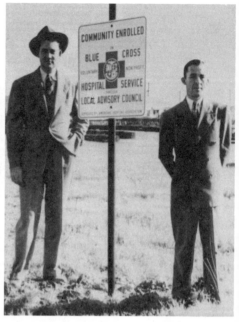

Community enrollment in Gainesville, 1940s

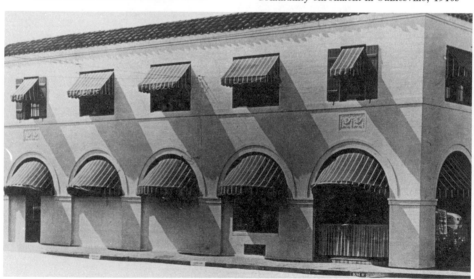

The building at Bryan and Olive was GHS's home from 1940 to 1946.

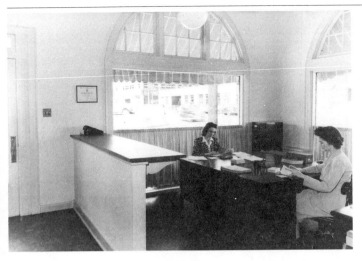

Life at Bryan and Olive:

The entrance and reception area. Euline Mitchell, right, was receptionist and public relations director. Dorothy Rambo managed individual enrollment.

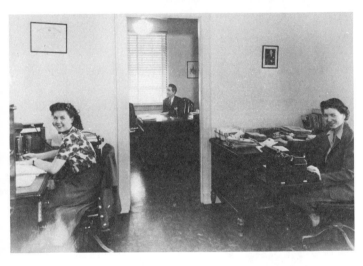

Assisting McBee were Patty Dague, left, and Annie Laurie Surratt.

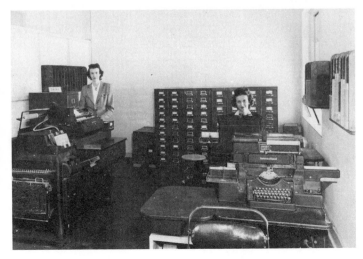

Olga Sykes, left, managed the electrical accounting machines, assisted by Helen Thompson.

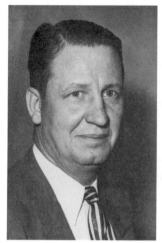

Harley B. West, director of
enrollment

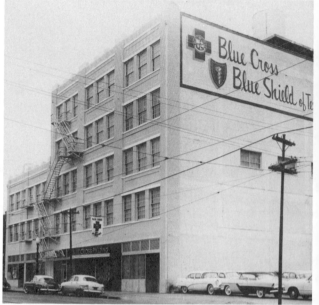

The building at 2208 Main was renovated from an auto pound and
was the company's home from 1946 to 1960.

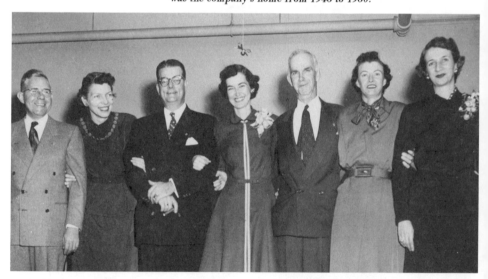

At the Christmas party in 1951, these employees each celebrated 10 years with the company: George
Dorsa, Annie Laurie Surratt, Ned Prigmore, Euline Mitchell, Kenneth Dealey, Olga Sykes, Helen
Thompson.

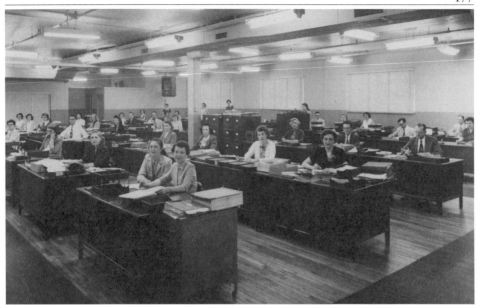

1953 employees pause for the photographer

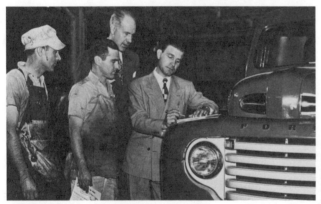

Ford employees in Texas added the new Blue Shield benefits to their coverage, 1949.

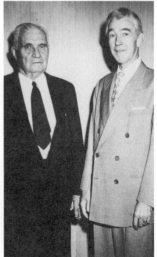

McBee and Kimball, 1954

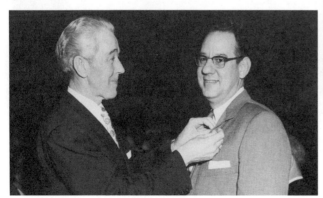

Tom Beauchamp receives his 10-year service pin from McBee, 1954.

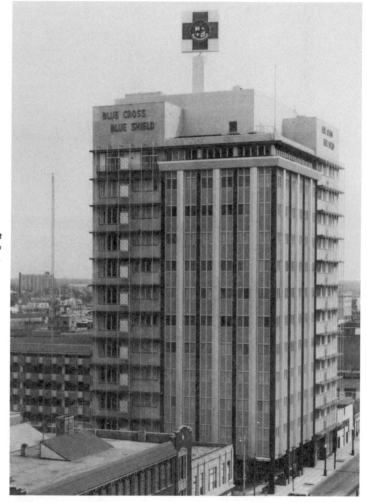

The symbol of pride. It served as headquarters from 1960 to 1980.

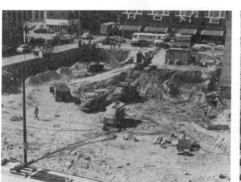

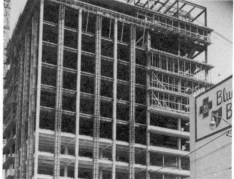

From their vantage point across the street, employees viewed the building progress. Left, 1958; right, 1959.

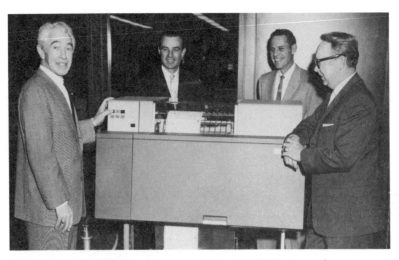

The printer of the IBM 1401, the company's first (and Dallas' second) computer.
Left to right, McBee, Gene Aune, Frank Henry, Bob Bourland, 1962.

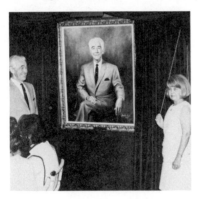

Lillian McBee unveils the portrait of her
husband, 1967.

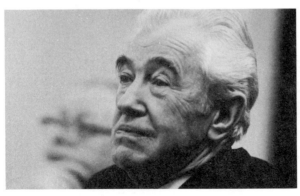

McBee shortly before
his death, 1967.

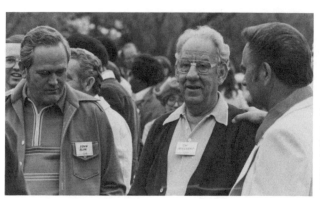

Beauchamp with longtime sales professionals Erwin Blum and
Howard Craft at the 1978 state sales meeting.

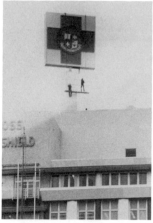

Workers begin the arduous task
of changing the rotating cross
from the AHA insignia to the
new look, 1974.

Tom Beauchamp guided the
company through many changes.

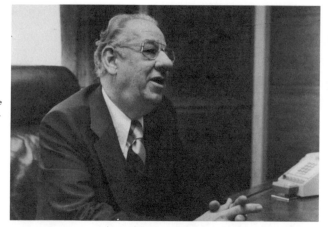

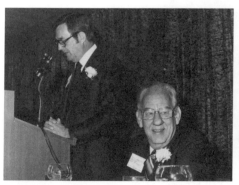

At his 1978 retirement dinner, Beauchamp enjoys
some good-natured ribbing from incoming
president Walt Hachmeister.

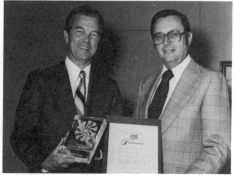

Hachmeister and Dallas mayor Robert Folsom
who proclaimed April 19, 1979, as Blue Cross
Day in Dallas in honor of 50 years of service.

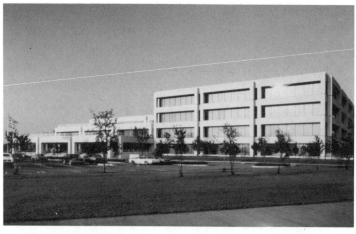

The Richardson building provided much-needed space for the company when it was finished in 1980.

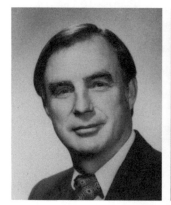

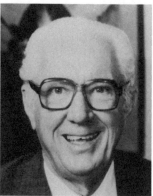

Acting President Gene Aune

Board Chairman John Justin who enticed Melton out of retirement

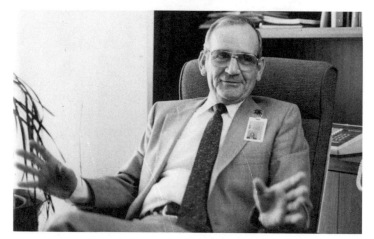

John Melton rescued the company during critical times.

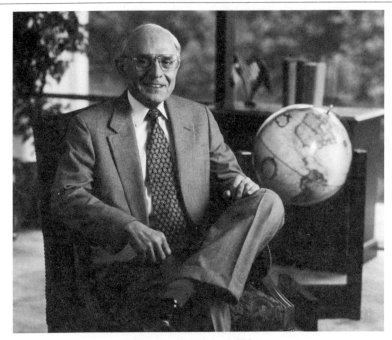

Rogers K. Coleman, M.D.
"Stronger together" became a familiar phrase as the Texas and Illinois Plans merged their strengths into a regional enterprise.

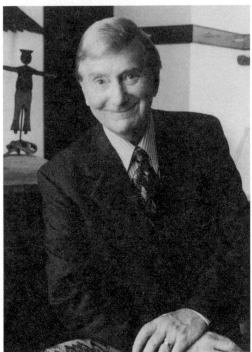

Ray McCaskey

Members of the Boards of Directors

Group Hospital Service, Inc./ Blue Cross and Blue Shield of Texas, Inc.

Group Medical and Surgical Service

Group Life and Health Insurance Company

Name	Title	Period Served
J. H. Groseclose	Chm. & Pres. (5/39 - 8/39 & 2/40 - 5/43)	5/39-1943
L. N. Markham, M.D.	Vice President ('39-'50)	5/39-1951
Josie M. Roberts	Secy.- Treas. ('39-'41), 2nd VP ('47-'50)	5/39-1953
C. E. Hunt		5/39-1945
Ara Davis		5/39-10/39
Martha Roberson		5/39-1940
Margaret Hales Rose	Secy. ('41-'46)	5/39-1946
Robert Jolly	2nd VP ('43-'46)	8/39-1946
Lucius R. Wilson, M.D.	Chm. & Pres. (8/39–2/40)	8/39-1941
John F. Donohoe		10/39-1940
E. H. Cary, M.D.	Treas. ('42-'43), Pres. ('43-'53)	10/39-1953
George B. Dealey		10/39-1946
Preston Hunt, M.D.		10/39-1942
John H. Burleson, M.D.	Honorary Lifetime Director	10/39-1953
Leslie Hogan		10/39-1942
J. P. McCord		11/39-1942
Earl M. Collier	Treas. ('57-'67), Honorary Lifetime Director	1940-1971
E. O. Nichols, M.D.		1941-1942
Harry G. Hatch		1942-1947
Judson Taylor, M.D.		1942-1943
Ben Taub		1942-1947
Charles F. Ashcroft		1940-1946
J. Anderson Fitzgerald, Ph.D.		1943-1950
J. Howard Payne	Treas. ('43-'53)	1942-1954
Alfreda P. Hassell		1943-1950
Sister Mary Vincent		1943-1947
Tol Terrell	1st VP ('50-'52), 2nd VP ('53-'55), Treas. ('67-'77), Honorary Lifetime Director	1943-1977
Lawrence Payne	Secy. ('46-'52), 1st VP ('52), Treas. ('53)	1943-1954
W. E. Justin		1943-1948
M. J. Norrell	Secy. ('52-'57), Honorary Lifetime Director	1943-1960
Chauncey D. Leake, Ph.D.		1944-1955
George R. Enloe, M.D.*		1945-1949
J. Charles Dickson, M.D.*		1945-1954
B. E. Pickett, Sr., M.D.*	Honorary Lifetime Director	1945-1956
F. T. McIntire, M.D.*		1945-1947
H. F. Connally, M.D.		1945-1948
E. A. Rowley, M.D.	2nd VP (3/64 – 9/64), Pres. (9/64 - 4/65), Honorary Lifetime Director	1945-1970
C. J. Hollingsworth	Honorary Lifetime Director	1945-1973
Wayne J. Holmes		1946-1952
Eva M. Wallace		1947-1953
L. H. Allen	Treas. ('54), 1st VP ('55 – '57), Pres. ('57-'64)	1947-1964
John G. Dudley	1st VP ('54), 2nd VP ('55-'64), Honorary Lifetime Director	1947-1964
Olin Culberson		1947-1954
J. Walter Hammond	Honorary Lifetime Director	1947-1960
Sister Alberta	2nd VP ('50)	1947-1954
Robert B. Homan, Jr., M.D.		1948-1961
F. J. L. Blasingame, M.D.	1st VP ('53), Pres. ('54-'57)	1948-1957

Louis C. Heare, M.D.*		1949-1952
Allen T. Stewart, M.D.*		1949-1961
Taylor Glass		1950-1953
J. F. Morrison		1950-1954
Carroll H. McCrary	Honorary Lifetime Director	1951-1975
Waldo Bernard		1952-1955
Denton Kerr, M.D.*	Honorary Lifetime Director	1953-1973
Dunbar Chambers		1953-1956
Albert H. Scheidt	Treas. ('55-'57)	1953-1965
Everett C. Fox, M.D.	Secy. ('57-'71), Honorary Lifetime Director	1953-1971
Max Clampitt		1954-1957
J. B. Copeland, M.D.	Honorary Lifetime Director	1954-1965
R.W. Kimbro, M.D.*		1954-1969
F. S. Walters, Jr.		1954-1963
Burton Sears		1954-1956
Sister Mary Helen		1954-1961
W. P. Earngey, Jr.	Honorary Lifetime Director	1955-1976
F. R. Weddington		1955-1957
Walter E. Long	Honorary Lifetime Director	1955-1967
J. Elro Brown		1955
Harvey Renger, M.D.	Honorary Lifetime Director	1956-1978
Howard T. Tellepsen		1957-1960
James W. Aston	1st VP ('58-'65), Pres./Chm. ('65-'78), Chm. Emeritus ('78), Honorary Lifetime Director	1957-1978
Boone Powell, Sr.	Secy. ('71-'76), Honorary Lifetime Director	1957-1976
Tom B. Bond, M.D.*		1958-1963
D. B. (Pete) Campbell	Honorary Lifetime Director	1958-1975
L. A. Sunkel		1960-1963
L. J. Whetsell	1st VP ('65-'69), Honorary Lifetime Director	1960-1969
J. H. West		1960-1968
Robert H. Bell, M.D.*		1961-1965
Olin B. Gober, M.D.*		1961-1972
Horace M. Cardwell	Treas. ('77-'80), Lifetime Director Emeritus	1962-1995
C. H. DeVaney		1963-1968
James A. Hallmark, M.D.*	Lifetime Director Emeritus	1963-1988
John S. Justin, Jr.	2nd VP ('65-'69), 1st VP ('69-'78), Chm. ('78-'85), Chm. Emeritus ('85-'98), Lifetime Director Emeritus	1963-1998***
Sister Elizabeth		1963-1969
W. Wilson Turner	Honorary Lifetime Director	1964-1981
William L. Lindholm		4/65 - 7/65
Alvin W. Bronwell, M.D.ˀ		1965-1971
Robert F. Gossett, M.D.		1965-1977
T. Henry Morrison, Jr.		1965-1977
E. C. (Ted) Smith		1967-1968
Robert B. Cullum	2nd Vice Chm. ('70-'78), 1st Vice Chm. ('78-'81)	1967-1981
Louis C. Bailey	2nd Vice Chm. ('69-'70)	1968-1970
Sidney Dean		1968-1971
Harry Peterson		1968-1979
Sister Marie Breitling		1969-1975
Charles B. Dryden, Jr., M.D.	Lifetime Director Emeritus	1969-1998***
Charles Max Cole, M.D.	Secy. ('76-'80), Lifetime Director Emeritus	1970-1998***
Walter A. Brooks, M.D.		1971-1980
Joseph T. Painter, M.D.*		1971-1980

J. T. (Red) Woodson		1971-1975
Arthur L. McElmurry		1971-1980
Ellis Campbell, Jr.		1972-1981
Bill E. Collins	2nd Vice Chm. ('78-'82), 1st Vice Chm. ('82-'85), Chm. ('85-'97), Chm. Emeritus ('97), Lifetime Director Emeritus	1972-1997
James H. Sammons, M.D.*		1972-1974
James A. Robinson		1973-1977
Joseph T. Ainsworth, M.D.*		1974-1979
Mario E. Ramirez, M.D.		1974-1993
L. M. Kennedy, D.D.S.	Lifetime Director Emeritus	1974-1998
Carrol G. Chaloupka	Lifetime Director Emeritus	1975-1991
George B. Pearson	Lifetime Director Emeritus	1975-1998***
Sister Louise Scheessele		1975-1977
R. J. Christie		1975-1976
Guy H. Dalrymple	Lifetime Director Emeritus	1976-1994
Boone Powell, Jr.		1976-1977
Doyle E. Rogers		1977-1985
Sam D. Young, Jr.		1977-1981
E. D. (Don) Walker		1977-1978
Joe B. Rushing, Ph.D.	1st Vice Chm. ('90-'97), Chm. ('97-'98) Lifetime Director Emeritus	1978-1998
Marcella D. Perry		1978-1982
John M. Smith, Jr., M.D.	Lifetime Director Emeritus	1978-1998***
Tom L. Beauchamp, Jr.*		9/78 -12/78
Walter F. Hachmeister*		1979-1981
Dan E. Butt	Lifetime Director Emeritus	1979-1996
James L. Jones	Chm., Texas Affiliate Board ('99), Lifetime Director Emeritus	1979-1998***
W. Clay Ellis	Lifetime Director Emeritus	1980-1998
J. Liener Temerlin		3/81 -10/81
Alton Pearson		1981-1986
Eugene W. Aune*		3/81 -10/81
John D. Melton*	Chm. (5/85), Lifetime Director Emeritus	1981-1990
W. C. (Bill) Hatfield		1982-1992
John Ben Shepperd	1st Vice Chm. ('85-'90), Lifetime Director Emeritus	1982-1990
Jack A. Griggs, Ph.D.		1983-1998**
James R. Adams		1984-1988
William P. Daves, Jr.*		5/85
Ray Farabee	1st Vice Chm. ('97-'98)	1989-1998**
Tieman H. ("Skipper") Dippel, Jr.		1989-1998**
M. Ray Perryman, Ph.D.		1990-1998***
Rogers K. Coleman, M.D.*		1991-1998**
Maria Elena A. Flood		1993-1998**
Ross B. Snyder*		1993-1998
Milton Carroll		1994-1998**
Patsy B. Leins*		1998-

* Director of Group Medical and Surgical Service and/or Group Life and Health Insurance Company only.

** Member of Health Care Service Corporation (HCSC) Board of Directors representing Blue Cross and Blue Shield of Texas effective 1/1/99 following the merger of the two companies 12/31/98.

*** Member of Texas Affiliate Board of HCSC effective 1/1/99 following the merger of the two companies 12/31/98.

Presidents

Group Hospital Service, Inc. / Blue Cross and Blue Shield of Texas, Inc.
1939-1998

Bryce Twitty	Administrator	July 1, 1939 - August 10, 1940
Justin Ford Kimball	Administrator	August 15, 1940 - August 15, 1941
Walter R. McBee	Administrator Executive Director President (Named inabsentia on August 28, 1967, died August 30, 1967)	August 15, 1941 June 19, 1945 April 8, 1967
Tom L. Beauchamp, Jr.	Interim CEO President	August 28, 1967 March 15, 1968 - December 31, 1978
Walter F. Hachmeister	President	January 1, 1979 - March 27, 1981
Eugene W. Aune	Acting President	March 27, 1981 - October 19, 1981
John D. Melton	President	October 19, 1981 - April 30, 1985
William P. Daves, Jr.	President	May 1, 1985 - May 31, 1985
John D. Melton	President	May 31, 1985 - December 31, 1990
Rogers K. Coleman, M.D.	President	January 1, 1991 - December 31, 1998

Health Care Service Corporation
January 1, 1999 to present

Ray McCaskey	President and CEO Illinois Division President
Rogers K. Coleman, M.D.	Texas Division President Chairman of the Board

Notes

Chapter One: **The Man and the Formula**

1. Kimball, interview with Munn.
2. Rose-Mary Rumbley, *A Century of Class: Public Education in Dallas 1884-1984.* (Austin: Eakin Press, 1984), 92.
3. Kimball, interview with Munn.
4. Ibid.
5. *Dallas Morning News*, March 10, 1952. This story reported on him revising his 1924 history in 1952.
6. Quoted in Lana Henderson, *Baylor University Medical Center: Yesterday, Today and Tomorrow* (Waco: Baylor University Press, 1978), 71.
7. For a general discussion of the metamorphosis of the modern hospital industry, see "The Reconstitution of the Hospital" in Starr, *The Social Transformation of American Medicine*, 145-179.
8. *Daily Times Herald* (Dallas), June 8, 1929. Despite the hopes of those who assembled that evening, Baylor College of Medicine was not to find a permanent home in Dallas. Funding for the medical college had long been an issue, and in 1939 the Southwestern Medical Foundation was created to offer a better funding base. The foundation also insisted that the medical college become non-sectarian and not be controlled by the Baptists. Tensions increased between the foundation and the college until the college moved to Houston in 1943. In part, it was lured by a lucrative offer from M.D. Anderson Foundation, and in part it was trying to stay in the Baptist and Baylor University fold. Southwestern Medical College was then founded, which remains in Dallas as part of the University of Texas system. Baylor's School of Pharmacy closed in 1931; the dental and nursing schools remain active.
9. Kimball, interview with Munn.
10. Starr, *The Social Transformation of American Medicine*, 241-242.
11. Kimball, interview with Munn.
12. Kimball letter to Dallas school teachers, 1929.

Chapter Two: **Selling the New Idea**

1. Kimball, interview with Munn.
2. Ibid.
3. Ibid.
4. Twitty, interview with Munn.
5. Marian Green, statement given January 20, 1954, Dallas.
6. Payne, interview with Munn.
7. Ibid.
8. Kimball, interview with Munn.
9. Undated newspaper clipping.
10. *Dallas Morning News*, February 13, 1954.
11. Kimball, interview with Munn.
12. For a general discussion of the rise of the medical profession, see Starr, *The Social Transformation of American Medicine*, 290-334.
13. Kimball, interview with Munn.
14. Payne, interview with Munn.
15. Ibid.

16. Twitty, interview with Munn.

17. Van Dyk, interview with Munn.

18. Ibid.

19. Ibid.

20. Van Steenwyk, interview with Fairbairn.

21. Cunningham and Cunningham, *The Blues: A History of the Blue Cross and Blue Shield System*, 17-33.

22. Lawrence Payne, "The Birth of Blue Cross and My Early Connection With It," standard speech presented to hospital administrative residents at Baptist Memorial Hospital in Jacksonville, Florida, from 1963 to 1970.

PART TWO: THE STORY OF BLUE CROSS AND BLUE SHIELD OF TEXAS

Chapter Three: Shaky Beginnings

1. "Medical Profession, Its Composite Character and Relationships," *Texas State Journal of Medicine*, February 1932.

2. Ibid.

3. *Dallas Morning News,* Dec. 21, 1934.

4. *Fort Worth Star-Telegram,* April 22, 1939, and minutes of the tenth annual THA Assembly, Fort Worth.

5. According to a July 7, 1976, memo from company attorney Steve G. McDonald to Harley B. West, two other companies were later organized under the original enabling status. East Texas Group Hospitalization System, Inc. was granted a permit to organize on August 2, 1939, but was dissolved on November 10, 1949, by the State Board of Insurance after its liabilities had significantly exceeded assets. A second company, Fort Worth Negro Hospital Association, Inc., was granted a permit on April 19, 1941, but apparently the company never enrolled any members. It gave up the charter on August 27, 1943. A third entity was the Clinic Plan Service in Beaumont, which was chartered September 15, 1945, but later was reinsured into a company that became an insurance company.

6. Louis S. Reed, *Blue Cross and Medical Service Plans* (Washington, D.C.: Federal Security Agency, U.S. Public Health Service, 1947), pp. 18-20.

7. Twitty to Ernest Tennant, May 25, 1939.

8. Twitty to Markham, May 29, 1939.

9. Twitty to Groseclose, May 27, 1939.

10. Twitty to Hunt, May 26, 1939.

11. Twitty to Ford Motor Company, Dallas, June 15, 1939, and Lone Star Oldsmobile Company, Buick Motor Sales Corporation, and Dodge Manufacturing Corporation, Dallas, June 16, 1939.

12. *Dallas Morning News*, July 7, 1939.

13. Roberson to Twitty, June 12, 1939.

14. Twitty to Roberson, June 16, 1939.

15. Twitty to Jolly, October 2, 1939.

16. Twitty to Wilson, September 9, 1939.

17. Wilson to Twitty, September 12, 1939.

18. Groseclose to Jolly, August 14, 1939.

19. When GHS applied to the American Hospital Association in 1942, seeking approval as a Blue Cross Plan, the application shows the date of the company's first enrollment as July 25, 1939. The identity of the group is unknown.

20. Twitty to hospital superintendents, October 24, 1940.

21. Kimball's report to the GHS board of directors, February 8, 1941.

22. Rorem to Jolly, March 14, 1941.

23. Groseclose to Cary, May 30, 1941.

24. Report of McCarthy to GHS board of directors, June 1941.

Chapter Four: **Resetting the Foundation**

1. McBee to Overton, December 10, 1941.

2. *Advance*, November/December 1978.

3. Ibid.

4. McBee to Rorem, January 20, 1942.

5. Summary of meeting on May 25, 1956, with Ken Dealey, Annie Laurie Surratt, Olga Sykes, Helen Thompson and George Dorsa.

6. Ibid.

7. (Surratt) Drews, interview with author.

8. McBee to Overton, January 23, 1942.

9. McBee to Overton, December 30, 1941.

10. McBee to Rorem, February 13, 1942.

11. Groseclose to Critz, July 24, 1942.

Chapter Five: **Creating a Companion Company**

1. *Texas Blue Cross Bulletin*, August-September 1944.

2. Whit Plaisted to McBee, December 4, 1941.

3. McBee to Plaisted, December 11, 1941.

4. W. F. Dean to McBee, April 15, 1943.

5. McBee to Dean, April 16, 1943.

6. McBee to Rose, July 3, 1943.

7. McBee to F. M. Walters, June 23, 1943.

8. McBee to Terrell, February 8, 1944.

9. McBee to Dr. Connally, February 11, 1944.

Chapter Six: **Post-War Progress**

1. *Texas Blue Cross Bulletin*, September 1946.

2. "Blue Cross Day Idea Draws Quick A. & H. Protest" in *The Insurance Record for The Southwest Insurer*, April 1947.

3. Booth Mooney, *More Than Armies: The Story of Edward H. Cary, M.D.* (Dallas: Mathis Van Nort & Co., 1948), iv. Mathis Van Nort & Co. was the publishing company owned by the grandfather of longtime Blue Cross and Blue Shield of Texas employee Marilyn M. Mathis.

4. Cunningham and Cunningham, *The Blues: A History of the Blue Cross and Blue Shield System*, 75.

5. McBee to board of directors, June 5, 1946.

6. West, untitled history, chapter five, 4-5.

7. Cunningham and Cunningham, *The Blues: A History of the Blue Cross and Blue Shield System*, 61.

8. McBee, "Report and Recommendations to the Board of Directors," July 24, 1947.

Chapter Seven: **The Maturing of the Company**

1. West to enrollment departments, December 16, 1954.
2. *Dallas Morning News*, January 6, 1952.
3. *Waco Times Herald,* October 9, 1956.
4. West to area office department heads, April 21, 1950.
5. Attachment to letter from McBee to board members, March 19, 1953.

Chapter Eight: **A Living Symbol**

1. Beauchamp to McBee, July 25, 1957.
2. Hahn, interview with author.
3. Johnson, interview with author.
4. Ibid.
5. Walters, interview with author.
6. Bourland to McBee, December 5, 1960.
7. McBee to Beauchamp, January 9, 1961.

Chapter Nine: **Exponential Growth**

1. Beauchamp to McBee, August 29, 1961.
2. Aune, interview with author.
3. Ibid.
4. Buzbee, interview with author.
5. Beauchamp to West, November 13, 1961.
6. Radio script, November 1961.
7. West to sales and executive staff, August 17, 1962.
8. West to enrollment personnel, October 20, 1965.
9. Minutes of the GHS board meeting, April 10, 1965.
10. McBee, "State of the Plan, 1966" given to the board of directors, undated.
11. Quoted in Cunningham and Cunningham, 159.
12. Harvey, interview with author.
13. (Fischer) Wright, interview with author.
14. McBee, speech to the House of Delegates of the Texas Hospital Association, May 16, 1965.
15. Aune, interview with author.
16. Ibid.

Chapter Ten: **The Challenges of Change**

1. West to executive and marketing staff, November 21, 1968.
2. Beauchamp, address to the board of directors, March 31, 1973.
3. Ibid.
4. Beauchamp, address to the board of directors, September 27, 1973.
5. Beauchamp, address to the board of directors, September 28, 1974.
6. Beauchamp, address to the board of directors, March 25, 1972.
7. Beauchamp, address to the board of directors, March 30, 1974.
8. Aune, interview with author.
9. Beauchamp, cited in *Advance*, October 1978.

Chapter Eleven: **Taking Risks**

1. Hachmeister, cited in *Advance*, January 1979.
2. Hachmeister, address to the board of directors, March 31, 1979.
3. Hachmeister, cited in *Advance*, January 1980.
4. Hachmeister, interview with author.
5. Gwaltney, interview with author.
6. Minutes of the executive committee meeting, June 27, 1980.
7. Walker, interview with author.
8. Hachmeister, interview with author.
9. Aune, interview with author.
10. Hachmeister, interview with author.
11. Justin, interview with author.

Chapter Twelve: **Turnaround and Transition**

1. Justin, interview with author.
2. Melton, cited in *Advance*, December 1981.
3. *Dallas Morning News*, October 21, 1981.
4. Melton, cited in *Advance*, December 1981.
5. *Dallas Morning News,* December 30, 1981.
6. Colley, cited in *Advance*, April 1991.
7. Melton to all employees, March 1, 1982.
8. *Advance*, November 1984.
9. Melton, cited in *Advance,* April 1985.
10. Coleman, interview with author.

Chapter Thirteen: **Facing the Future**

1. Coleman, cited in *Advance*, April 1990.
2. Coleman, interview with author.
3. Ibid.
4. Coleman, executive office memorandum, August 31, 1993.
5. Coleman, cited in *Advances*, October 1994.
6. Coleman, executive office memorandum, September 13, 1994.
7. Coleman, executive office memorandum, March 23, 1995.
8. Coleman, interview with author.
9. Coleman, executive office memorandum, July 21, 1995.
10. Coleman, executive office memorandum, January 29, 1996.
11. Coleman, cited in *Advances*, October 1996.
12. Hall, cited in *now!*, February 1999. Employee newsletter.
13. Coleman, interview with author.

Primary Works

Blue Cross and Blue Shield of Texas, *Advance,* published 1976 to 1996. (Retitled *Advances* 1994 to 1996). Employee magazine.
_____. *Quota Busters,* published 1963 to 1983. Employee magazine.

Cunningham, Robert III and Robert M. Cunningham, Jr., *The Blues: A History of the Blue Cross and Blue Shield System.* DeKalb, Illinois: Northern Illinois University Press, 1997.

Fairbairn, Donald. Interview with E.A. van Steenwyk, Philadelphia, Pennsylvania, July 28, 1954. Tape recording, BCBSTX archives.

Munn, Melvin. Interview with Frank Van Dyk, Chicago, Illinois, July 23, 1954. Tape recording, BCBSTX archives.
_____. Interview with Justin Ford Kimball, Dallas, Texas, August 6, 1954. Tape recording, BCBSTX archives.
_____. Interview with Lawrence Payne, Tyler, Texas, August 19, 1954. Tape recording, BCBSTX archives.
_____.Interview with Bryce Twitty, Tulsa, Oklahoma, August 12, 1954. Tape recording, BCBSTX archives.

Schaal, Samuel. Interview with Eugene Aune, Richardson, Texas, October 18, 1996.
_____. Interview with Jack Buzbee, Richardson, Texas, January 12, 1999.
_____. Interview with Rogers K. Coleman, M.D., Richardson, Texas, May 28, 1999.
_____. Interview with Annie Laurie Drews, Dallas, Texas, February 11, 1999.
_____. Interview with Elaine Gwaltney, Dallas, Texas, May 17, 1999.
_____. Interview with Walter F. Hachmeister: Richardson, Texas, April 29, 1996; May, 6, 1996; May 15, 1996; May 20, 1996; May 29, 1996.
_____. Interview with E.W. Hahn, Richardson, Texas, November 26, 1996.
_____. Interview with Barbara Harvey, Richardson, Texas, April 14, 1999.
_____. Interview with Judy Johnson: Richardson, Texas, November 18, 1998; February 25, 1999.
_____. Interview with John Justin, Jr.: Richardson, Texas, May 22, 1996; Fort Worth, Texas, October 30, 1996.

_____. Interview with Vernon Walker, Richardson, Texas, February 17, 1999.

_____. Interview with George Walters, Richardson, Texas, March 24, 1999.

_____. Interview with Lelia Wright, Richardson, Texas, April 7, 1999.

Starr, Paul, *The Social Transformation of American Medicine.* New York: Basic Books, 1982.

West, Harley B., untitled and unpublished history of Blue Cross and Blue Shield of Texas, 1979.